WELCOME TO Sattvic Soul

EVERYDAY WELLNESS WISDOM

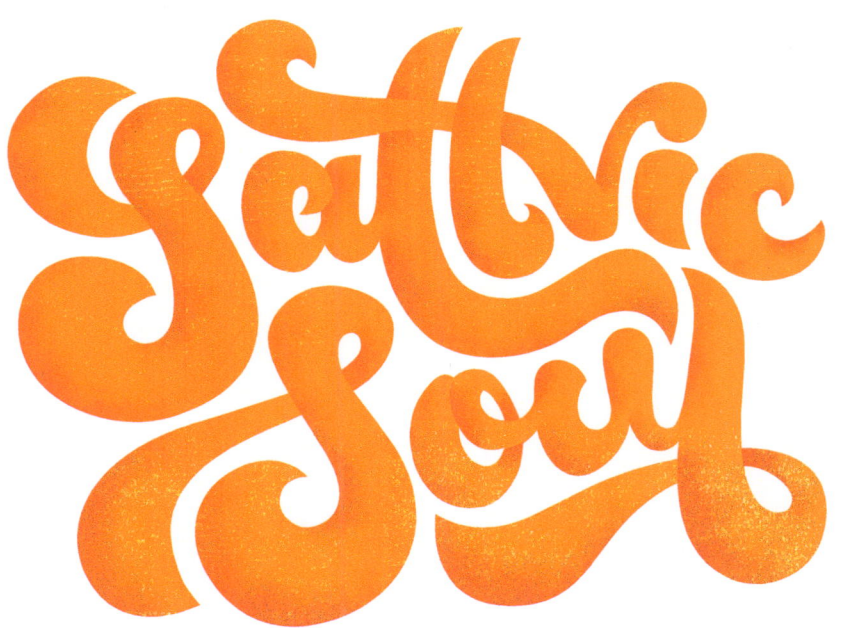

First published 2022

Copyright © Virginia Compton 2022

The right of Virginia Compton to be identified as the author of this work has been asserted in accordance with the Copyright, Designs & Patents Act 1988.

All rights reserved. No part of this book may be reproduced, stored in a retrieval system, or transmitted in any form or by any means, electronic, electrostatic, magnetic tape, mechanical, photocopying, recording or otherwise, without the written permission of the copyright holder.

Published under licence by Brown Dog Books and
The Self-Publishing Partnership Ltd, 10b Greenway Farm, Bath Rd, Wick, nr. Bath BS30 5RL

www.selfpublishingpartnership.co.uk

ISBN printed book: 978-1-83952-571-1

Cover and internal design by Sophie Maliphant

Illustrations by Sophie Maliphant and Ashma Dahal
Printed and bound in the UK
This book is printed on FSC® certified paper

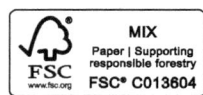

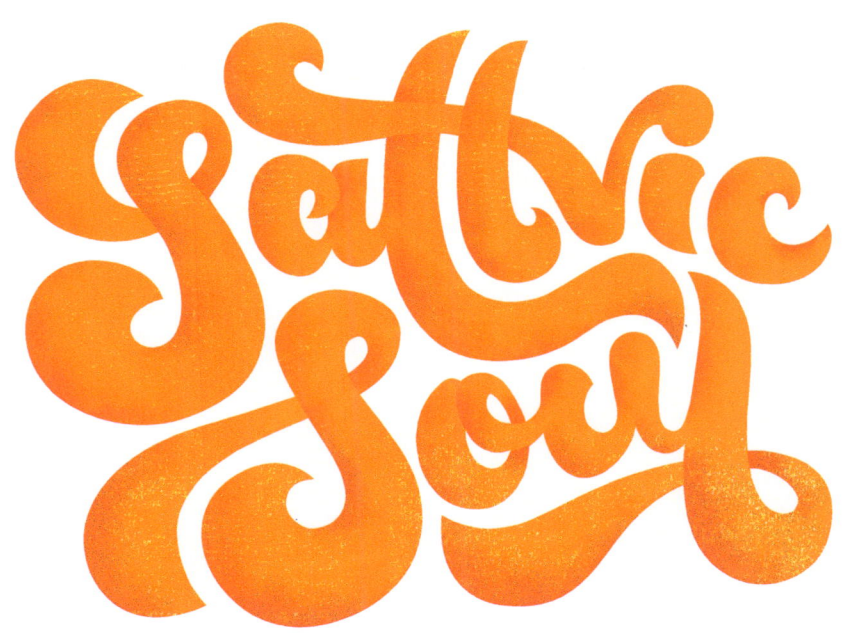

EVERYDAY WELLNESS WISDOM
VIRGINIA COMPTON

Illustrations by Sophie Maliphant and Ashma Dahal

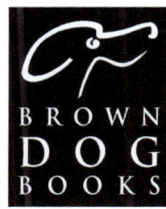

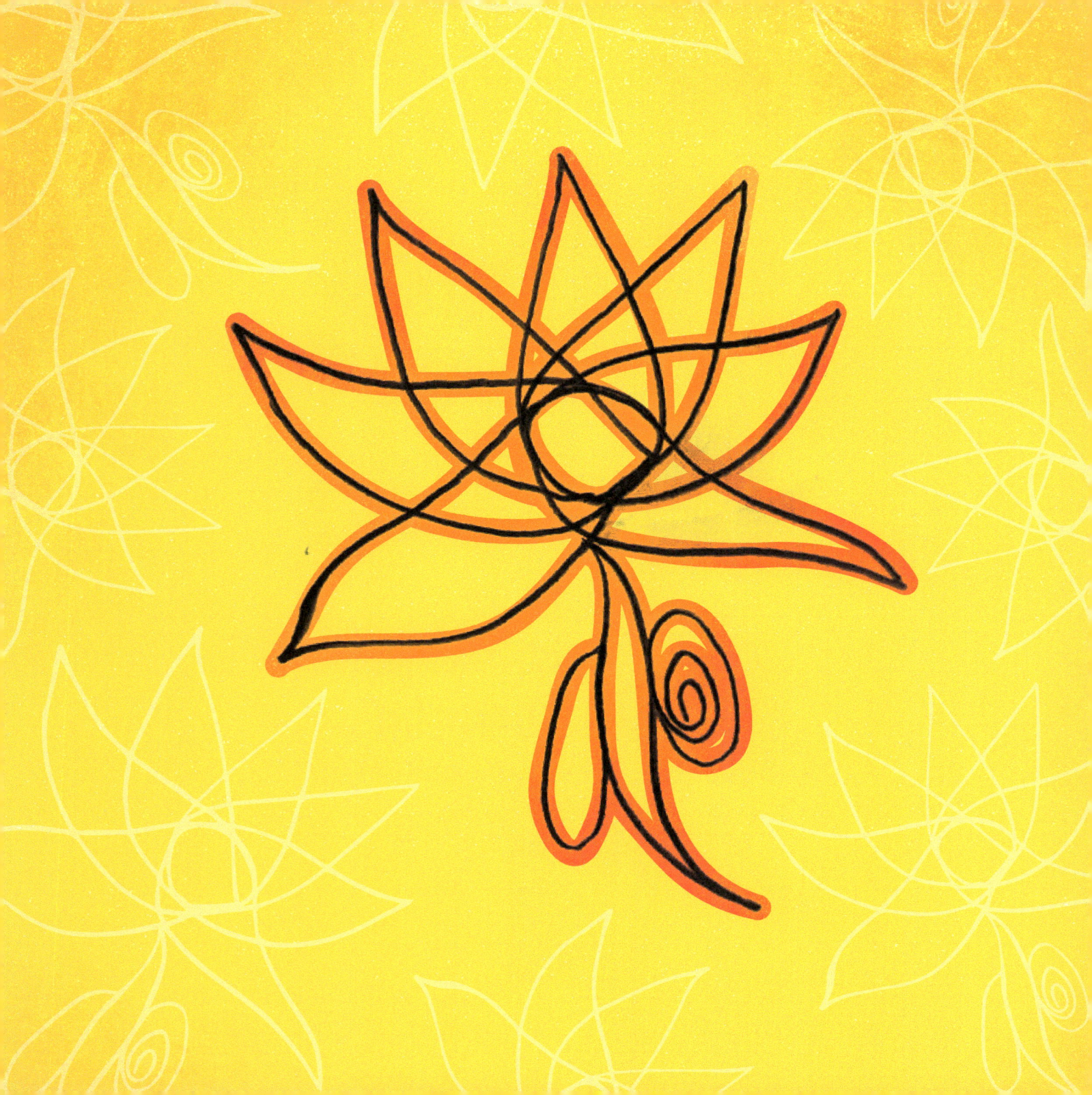

SATTVIC

To be in balance, to be healthy, happy, feeling at peace with a sense of harmony and well-being. This approach can apply to food, to ourselves in our body and mind or to our environment.

SOUL

Somehow we are aware that within us there is some kind of inner wisdom, a sense of knowing, an essence that reaches beyond the everyday.
This may be called the soul. The soul is always sattvic.

EVERYDAY WELLNESS WISDOM

This book shares a view of the world that is for everyday people, using the ancient wisdom of cycles and simple practices. This wisdom is an everyday thing. We can experience it in the cyclical nature of day and night, in our life cycle and beyond this into the cycles of the moon. We can embrace these cycles with awareness every day.

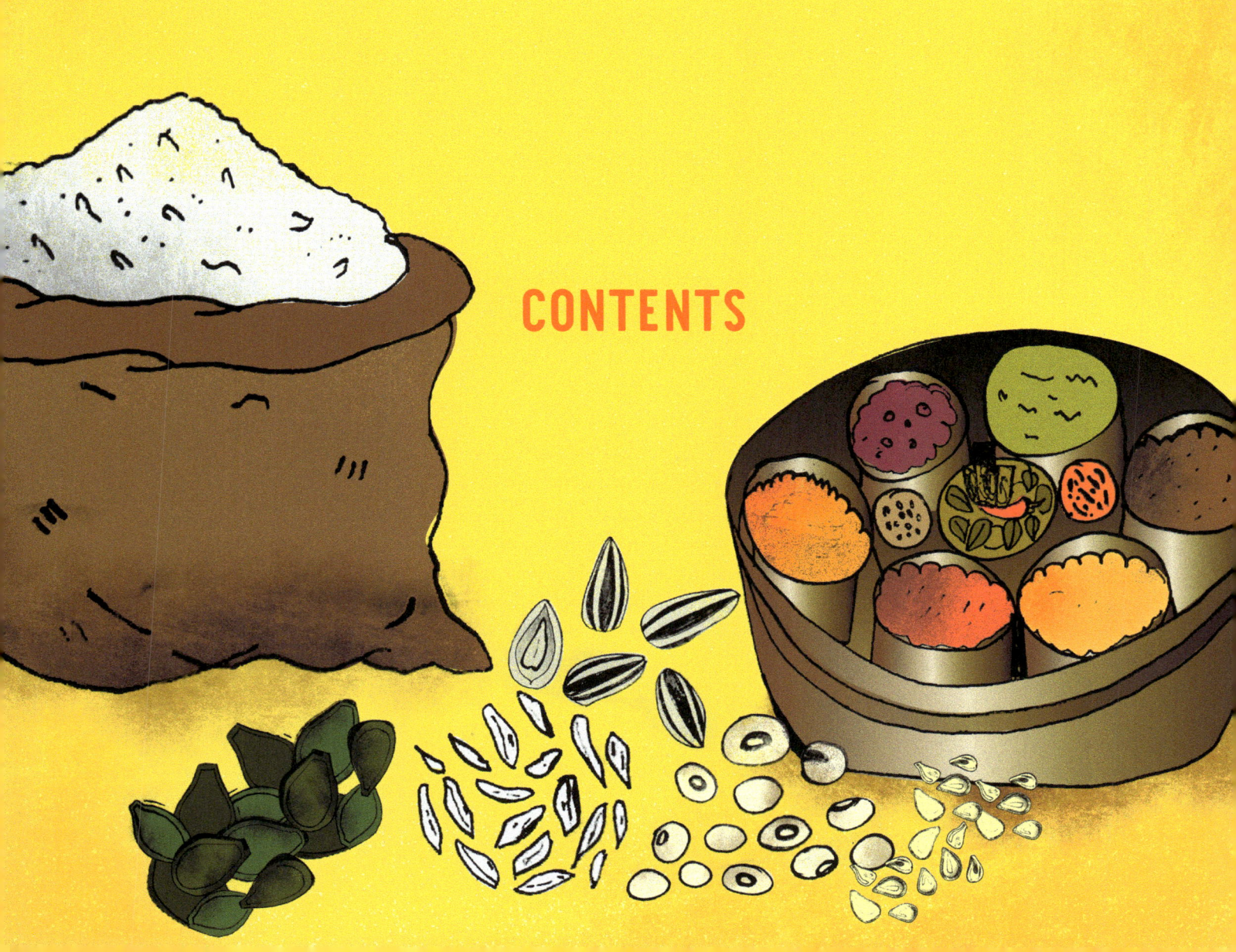

CONTENTS

FOREWORD
INTRODUCTION
page 13

LIFE IS A DANCE
page 18

GET IN TUNE WITH THE MOON
page 36

BECOMING SATTVIC
page 46

RECIPES
page 52

THE ISSUES ARE IN YOUR TISSUES
page 90

FASTING AND CLEANSING
page 99

THE JUICY STUFF
page 110

INGREDIENTS, EQUIPMENT AND COOKING NOTES
page 121

SATTVIC SOUL
page 128

GLOSSARY OF WORDS
page 132

RECIPES AND RITUALS INDEX
page 134

GRATITUDE
page 136

SUPPLIERS, SERVICES AND CONNECTION
page 139

FOREWORD

In India every cow has its very own bird accompanying it.

The bird breed is a cattle egret.

It is a mutually beneficial relationship. The bird lives from the bugs on the cow and the cow gets its bugs removed.

A fine example of how we should all care for one another.

Also maybe we can try to be our own egret sometimes, to look after ourselves, without questioning or analysing, just do what is good for us.

Be your own egret today and everyday.

Take extra special care of yourself.

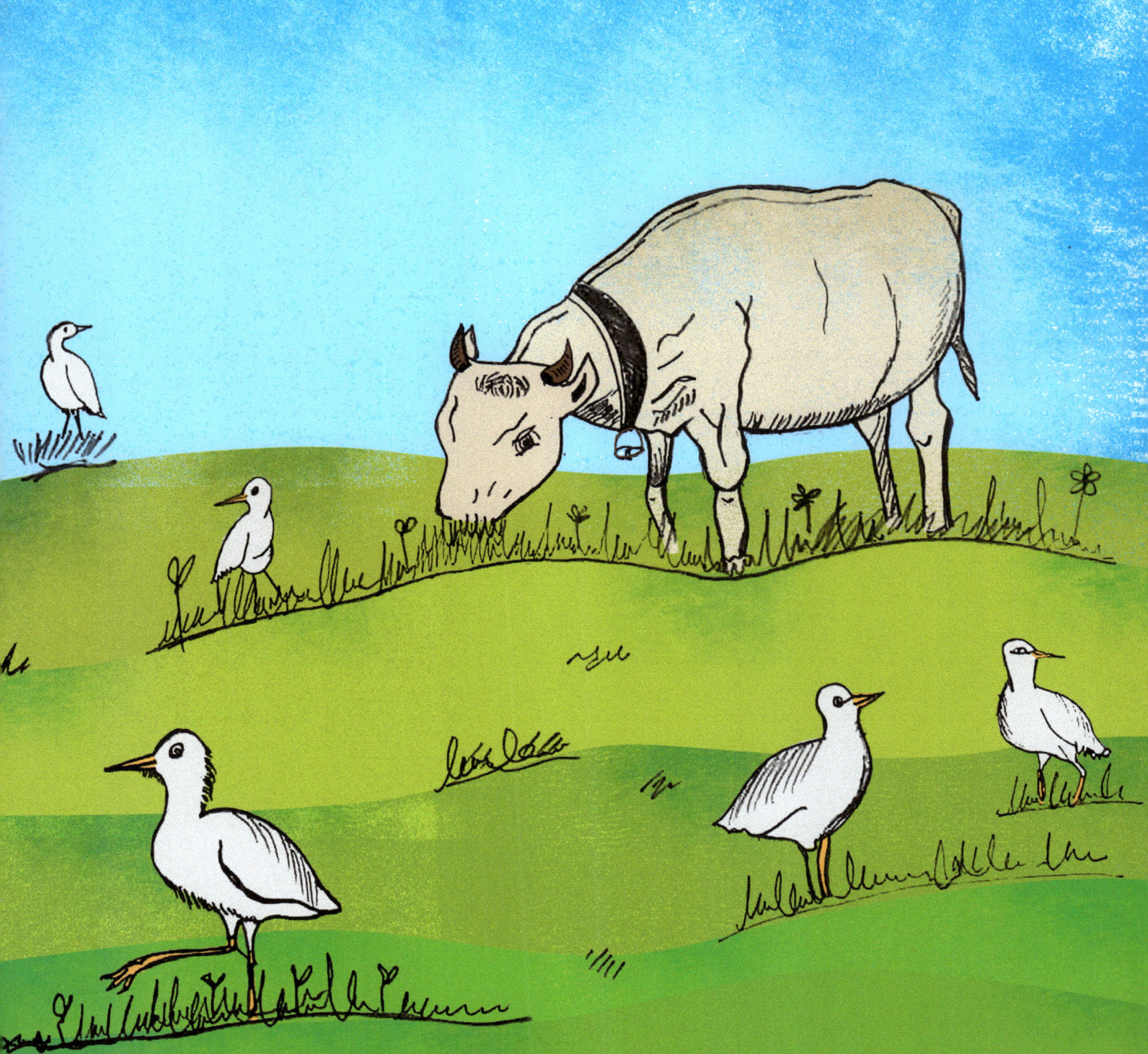

FOREWORD FROM SUNITA PASSI

Author, Ayurvedic Practitioner,
Founder Tri-Dosha Academy
UK | 2022

Virginia Compton walked through the doors of the Tri-Dosha Academy in October 2015 and I knew immediately I had met a kindred spirit. Having had an incredible experience of an Ayurvedic treatment in Kerala, India, Virginia had connected with the way I teach Ayurvedic bodywork to others beyond the level of technique. It soon became clear that her interest was in core principles, many of which are explored in concepts concerning the sattva. We have maintained a precious relationship ever since.

Before we met, Virginia had been a NHS level six nurse for most of her career. Interest in working with mental health and drug addiction changed her understanding of what health was: we are more than flesh and the influence of family and society. As her interest in spirituality and holistic medical care grew she found herself on the path I too was travelling. We're both passionate about providing people with ways to maintain not just their health, but a spiritual compass in a world of artificial stresses and pressures on our time, that impacts our hopes, our desire for a full life, and the sense that there may be more to existence.

The impact of social media and a celebrity-driven culture means we are deprived of soul nourishment and instead experience anxieties that only contemporary civilisation could have concocted. All of which helps explain the growing demand for ayurveda – and the beating heart at its core, knowledge and experience of the gunas, which is where sattva can be found. The good news is, you've been there already...

Step out of the hurly-burly of everyday life - temporarily even, which is as good as it gets frankly - and you'll begin to notice the different forces pushing and pulling at your attention can be considered as (broadly speaking) active and passionate, chaotic and sometimes destructive, or serene and balanced. They can form an unmerry-go-round at times, awareness of which can help spend your time on it more effectively. And there's the prospect with that of existing more in the calm harmonious space called sattva.

A woman gifted with healing hands and a formidable energy, Virginia will help you unravel this ancient knowledge accumulated over her lifetime of curiosity. She is the bridge between West and East. A nurse turned ayurveda practitioner, her insight provides a radically different mindset than the West's 'magic bullet' approach and gives us more confidence in our own ability to heal ourselves, exercising discernment and focusing on our greater potential gain.

Along the way, Virginia candidly shares very personal experiences, confidently wearing her heart on her sleeve, while she generously holds us and presents the invitation to do likewise to the extent that's right for us at this point. My deepest gratitude to Virginia - for penning these words, for going within to now help others, for knowing herself and purpose clearly with her graciousness and wisdom. I have been your teacher and you too are mine. It only remains for you - the reader - to enjoy these pages, learn from them, and discover how they begin to permeate your thoughts like the indefinably true scent of a rare flower, and be subtly reminded of it in the weeks ahead in your reflections, your feelings, your hopes and beliefs, and your new choices.

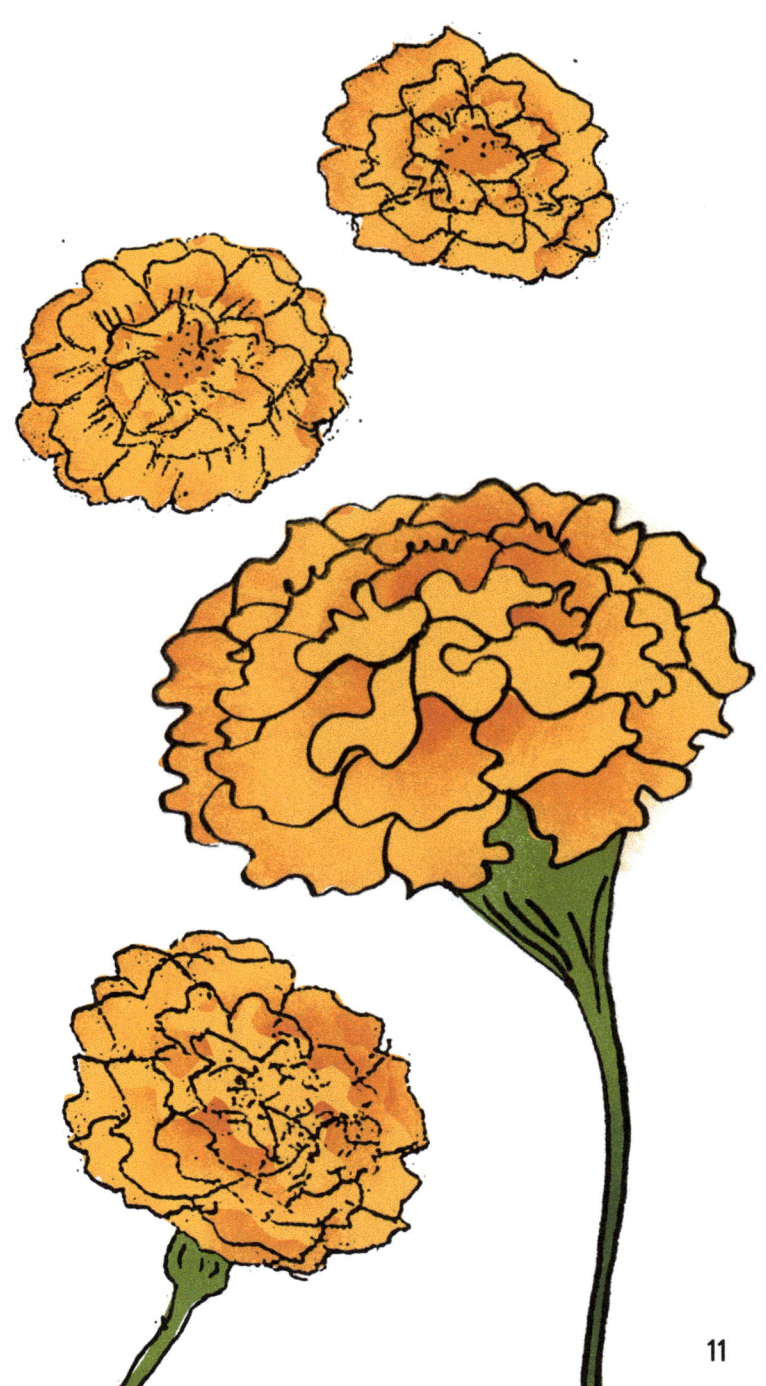

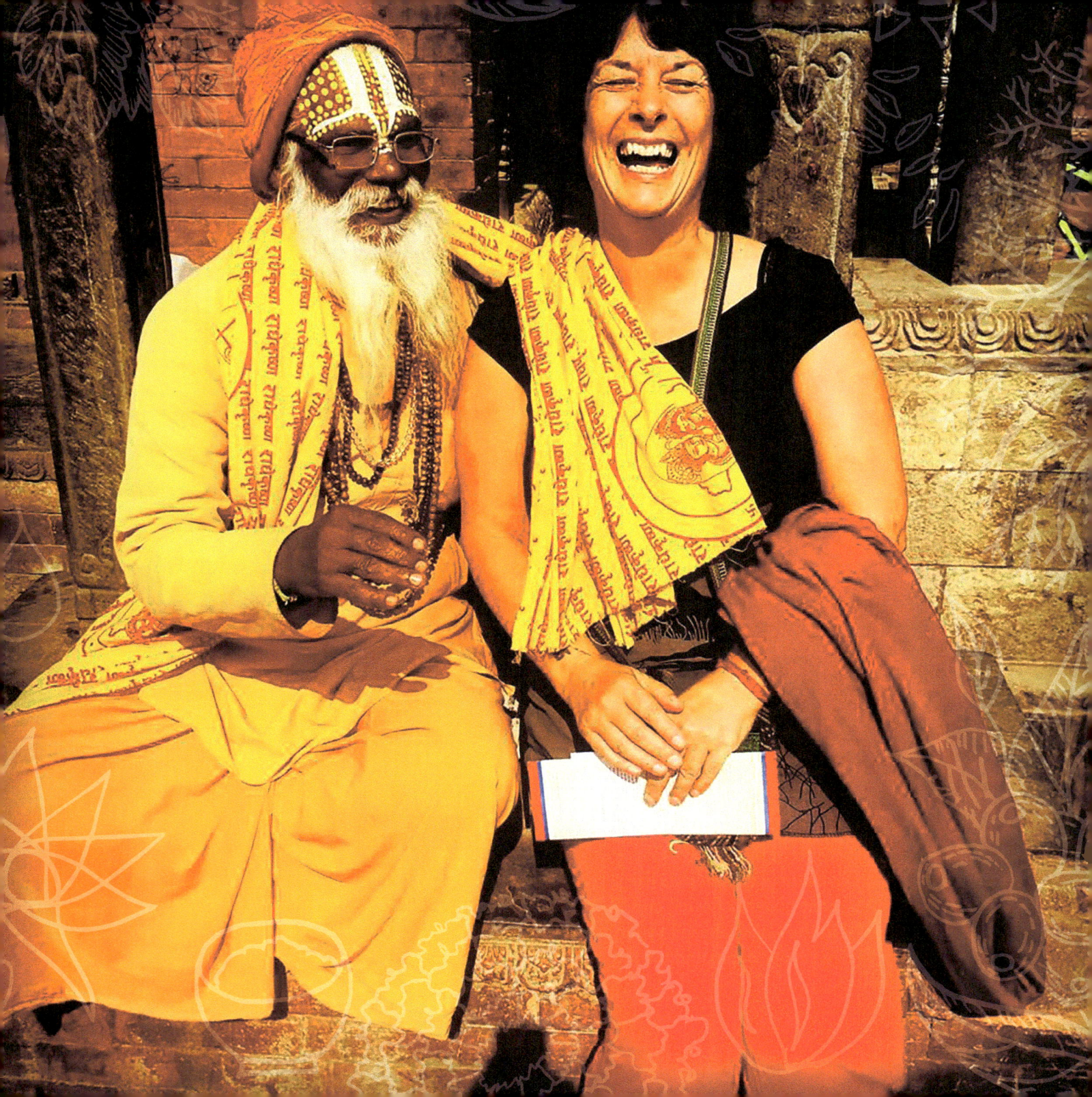

INTRODUCTION

This book is not a guide to ayurveda, or a description of yoga techniques. It is also not a recipe book. I draw upon the ancient principles and philosophies of ancient arts in order to offer a modern and do-able way of cyclical living that is in tune with nature, that brings about balance in the bodymind, and enables us to experience the sattvic soul.

Some words or terms as well as references to specific practices may be unfamiliar to you, please use the glossary and index at the back to check these out.

We are all responsible for ourselves. We can all take choices in how we live our lives, and therefore we can all choose, if we wish, to be healthy in terms of our food, lifestyle and general outlook on life. This approach to health and wellness is inspired by the tools and techniques of ayurveda, as well as cyclical wisdom and nature herself.

I recognise that some of you may already have some dis-ease or wonder how this approach can help you. To you I say, just give it a try, and see if making even a few simple changes in your daily habits, routine and lifestyle can shift things so you begin to feel 'better'. In my experience we often underestimate the healing effect of eating at a regular time, of going to bed in a routine and rhythmic manner and of allowing ourselves time and space to just be. I have witnessed great improvements for people who have adopted these simple daily practices.

The beauty of this system is that it is also largely free, and if not free then definitely fairly affordable. I have talked about keeping it affordable in the section on kitchen equipment and store cupboard ingredients and hope this feels helpful. This ancient wisdom is for everyone.

It is so easy to go with the flow. To live how your family or society expects you to live. To forget or push aside nature's rhythmic cycles and instead to not challenge or question anything, to eat the foods that are mainstream. To watch what everyone else watches on TV. To be caught up in the consumer society that feels so familiar and comfortable. This way of life no doubt gives a sense of security, safety and belonging to the majority, which is why most people may continue to live in this way. It is easier to go with the flow than to swim against the tide.

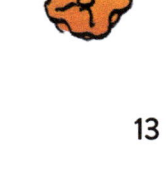

But is this the right thing for you? And is it really easier if it makes you unwell, physically and emotionally?

There is another way. A way that gives a real aliveness to our earthly existence. It is not always easy, and can be viewed as alternative, rebellious or just strange by the vast majority. But it will, even if embraced in part and definitely if taken in its entirety, give a vibrancy to life. A taste of what may be possible if we can be more true to ourselves. It can create a real feeling of physical and emotional strength and wellness in spite of what is happening in and around our individual experience. Wouldn't you rather reach your full potential, lie on your back in the wilderness and look at the stars, feeling vibrantly alive? You can truly experience what a thrill it is to feel that you have overcome adversity and you can choose to live your dreams. I believe that all humans have the potential to be truly amazing if they choose to be. It is not always easy, but it is absolutely possible.

This book is an offering of rituals and routines, food and recipes, cyclical wisdom and other thoughts that I wish to share with you. I hope it can help you along your journey to freedom. It is also practical, inexpensive in its suggestions and very real about our experience of everyday life. Come and join me.

BE THE CHANGE YOU WISH TO SEE IN THE WORLD.

Mahatma Gandhi

It may be helpful for you to know a little of my own journey. When we see someone living a life that is balanced, interesting, colourful it can be too easy to believe that this has always been the case. Oftentimes there is a journey, a story behind what you see on the surface.

As a child I hardly ever ate vegetables, and then only when forced. I really despised their taste, texture, colour, smell, everything about them. I also disliked 'PE' (physical education) as it was called. I found team games disheartening because I didn't feel like a team player, and lone sports, such as running, felt like torture. Emotionally and socially, I never particularly felt like I fitted in anywhere with anyone, this was exacerbated by the amount of times we moved house -every two or three years during my early years.

Fast forward to me now, aged 52 (at the time I am writing this) and I am an Ayurvedic Therapist, Yoga Teacher, Yoga Therapist and generally very enthusiastic about all things wellness related, especially healthy food and exercise. I feel confident when talking with other people, even complete strangers. I have lots of long-term friendships with amazing people in the local and global community. I generally feel very balanced, healthy and content in life. I feel I have really found my 'tribe' and my dharma (purpose) in life. Believe me when I say that, on a daily basis, I am amazed at where I find myself. It has been, and continues to be, an incredible and tumultuous journey, and it certainly didn't happen overnight.

DHARMA

Up until my early 30s I ate what you may call a regular western diet, meat, fish, dairy, eggs, vegetables, (some but not many more vegetables than when I was a child). I enjoyed alcohol, take away food, sugar and caffeine. Now I don't drink caffeinated drinks, I rarely eat chocolate, I avoid sugary foods, I don't eat meat. I only very occasionally eat dairy or oily fish, and I eat loads and loads of vegetables! How did I get here?

When I was growing up in 1970s Britain the diet was typically meat and vegetables, hot pots, Sunday roasts that kind of thing, puddings and cakes were relatively sugar laden and stodgy. Spaghetti bolognese was seen as very alternative and exotic! This way of eating had evolved from working on the land, and from the working classes of post war Britain, which is who my grandparents were. As society evolved we began to have a more sedentary work life so we didn't need this type of high carbohydrate energy laden food so much, but we continued to eat it anyway. We added in more 'exotic' things such as pasta, take away burgers and convenience foods or ready meals. As a teenager I lived with my dad. We survived on a particular brand of dried packet foods, I can recall now the powdery substance containing dried shrimps, the reconstituted 'beef', no fresh vegetables, and a treat was chips from the local Chinese takeaway.

I trained as nurse in the NHS in 1989. There was nothing on the training agenda about diet or nutrition whatsoever. Hospital food was notorious for being tasteless, bland and unappetising.

Now I look back with the benefit of hindsight, I wonder how anyone is supposed to heal and get well without good nutrition?

I first began to have my eyes opened by a boyfriend in 1992, he was particularly into cooking with spices and much more adventurous with food than anyone I had ever known. This is where I feel it all began. I began to notice that there is much more to food, and to life, much more than I had experienced to date. I became intrigued, curious, restless. I wanted and needed to learn more. I found a thirst for a knowledge of what it meant to be alive, to be a human, and everything this encompasses.

My life journey gradually continued and I explored and I discovered lots of different cultures, ways of viewing life as well as different foods. I was so delighted. I just knew there was so much more to explore! I always remember the experience and taste of my first butternut squash!

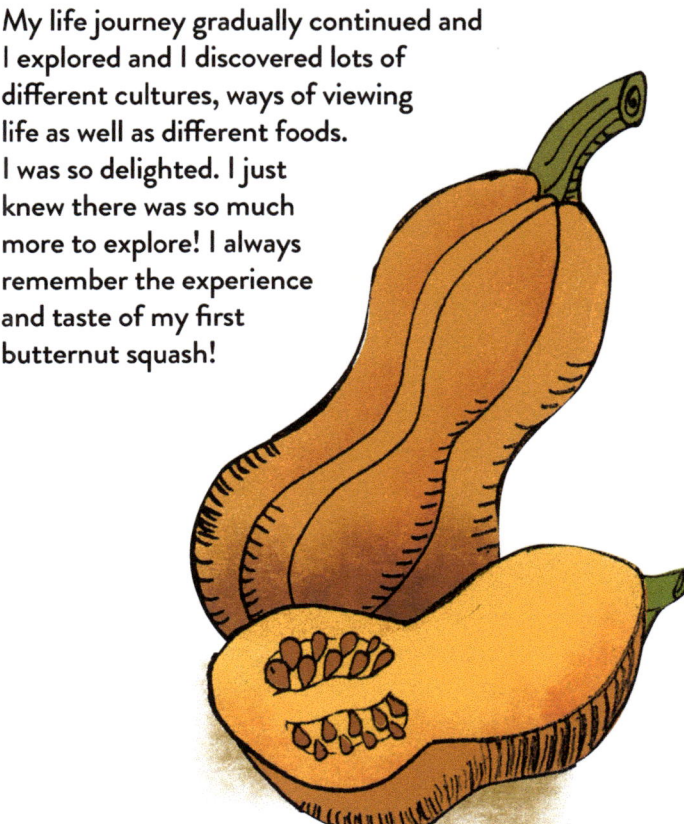

Now they are readily available, but I had not seen one until I started, around my early thirties, getting a veg box from a local farm. I was getting different vegetables each week and had to do something with them. I roasted the squash with red pepper and I had never tasted anything so delicious. Interestingly I only started getting the veg box because it was cheap. I couldn't afford very much meat, I had very little money, massive debts and was really struggling to survive psychologically and physically at that time. This in part is why I now feel you never can tell what you will learn and how you will grow from the life challenges you face. The veg box cost me £6 a week and then I had around £4 left, so £10 in total each week for food (in 2022 this would be around £20). This is why I know for sure that eating more healthily doesn't need to be very costly.

In 2003, after growing up in the midlands just south of Birmingham and then a few years in London, I moved to Devon, South West, UK. I still had very little in terms of money, but I had an optimism that was steadily building about how life could be. As soon as I arrived I noticed at a local church hall a beginners yoga course. I immediately enrolled. I didn't know anything about yoga, but instinctively felt like it was the right thing to do. I have not stopped practicing yoga since.

As a result of being in a more rural part of the world my life became more focused on the outdoors, and I embraced walking as a form of regular exercise, combining the physical activity with exploring and discovering all kinds of beautiful and interesting places, something I had already grown to love. I naturally began to enjoy physical activity, exertion and the way I felt during and afterwards. My energy levels and my psychological state improved as a result. It felt different to how PE felt at school because it was my choice and on my terms.

Whilst I was more active, studying yoga and living in a beautiful area I was still drinking alcohol, occasionally eating meat, drinking coffee, eating lots of sugar and chocolate. Like I said, this process didn't happen overnight. I noticed a few years in a row in the Autumn that I got a chesty cough. Always at the same time each year. This was a new thing from around the age of 35, and it happened four or five years in a row. The last couple of times it was a full blown chest infection and I was prescribed antibiotics from the GP. On the third time of seeing the GP I explained that I had noticed that this seemed to be a seasonal thing, this theory was dismissed out of hand. But I knew what I was experiencing so I researched some more. It was then I discovered ayurveda.

Ayurveda means science of life. It is a complete system for disease prevention. It is also used to treat diseases when they occur. This system is 5000 years old and originates from Kerala, South India. It is sometimes called the sister science of yoga. In ayurveda there are different body types or 'doshas'. My particular dosha, especially at that time, was very prone to 'damp' in the body, which can manifest as mucus, hence the chest infections. After a somewhat lengthy bargaining and debating process with myself I gave up dairy, which is incredibly mucus forming if that is your tendency. I have not had a chest infection since. I have become more and more involved over the years with the ayurvedic approach to health and wellness. I not only didn't get another chest infection, I lost a lot of body weight. I had eaten a lot of cheese in my lifetime and stopping this made an enormous difference.

I have gradually removed other things from my diet that don't suit my particular constitution. It's important to emphasise again that this is not an overnight process and it is definitely not a punitive thing. I notice each time I stop something that isn't helpful, it has a massively positive impact upon my physical and psychological health. My constitution has also continued to shift and change as I have aged, so my diet and lifestyle have been adapted accordingly and will continue to be. This may sound complex but it's really quite simple once you have a grasp of the basic principles. I have been incredibly fortunate to travel many times over the years to India, where ayurveda is an integral part of everyday life and the food there is naturally healthy and mostly vegetarian.

When my partner of 17 years died in 2017 my life completely fell apart. I lost our home, my business largely collapsed, I had absolutely, literally nothing left. The universe completely cleared me out. Ayurveda and yoga were all I had. At these times when life becomes so incredibly challenging these are the practices that can keep us going. This created a massive shift for me again, physically as well as emotionally. My coping strategies were definitely not always ideal. At that time, for a period of a couple of years, I returned to eating meat and drinking alcohol, and relying on caffeine, sugar and chocolate to artificially boost energy levels and to comfort myself. Food carries with it a great deal of emotional baggage. When we are under pressure, for whatever reason, this can be the most challenging time to stay focused on what is inherently good for us. Humans are complex and often illogical. Eventually, I got right back on the wagon in a bigger way than ever before.

I am sharing some of my story because I want you, dear reader, to know that I am speaking from my own personal experience and from my heart. It is all too easy to view someone sharing these foods, lifestyle and wellness practices as all perfect and totally together, but I do this because it keeps me sane. It keeps me healthy. I feel good when I do these things. I know who I am. It doesn't always make life easy and it certainly doesn't help you feel totally tranquil and enlightened! But it can definitely help you begin to feel good about yourself, and in my experience, that's a fine place to start.

In this book I am sharing rituals and recipes, cyclical wisdom and thoughts that I hope will be helpful for you, physically as well as psychologically, nurturing and nourishing your body, mind and sattvic soul.

THE UNIVERSE CLEARED ME OUT. AYURVEDA AND YOGA WERE ALL I HAD. WHEN LIFE BECOMES INCREDIBLY CHALLENGING THESE PRACTICES CAN KEEP US GOING.

Virginia Conran

LIFE IS A DANCE

Life is a dance
of elements
within and without
ourselves.
Spinning this way
and that
We can learn
to lean in
to become as one
with the mystery.

ELEMENTS, DOSHAS AND THE DAILY ROUTINE

One of the absolute cornerstones of wellness with ayurvedic principles is dinacharya, our daily self-care routine. In order to understand this it is first essential to get a basic understanding of the elements and different constitutional types. Of equal importance is the food we eat. If we eat food that is not suited to our body and our individual constitution this creates ama (meaning toxins) and eventually, if sustained over a prolonged period, this this will create inflammation and dis-ease.

Everything we experience and that exists is said to come from the five elements of earth, water, fire, air and ether. The food we eat is made of these elements and so are our bodies. In the kosha philosophy of yoga the body is called the 'anamaya kosha', meaning food body. We are literally what we eat. Food is our medicine, and it can heal or harm us.

The human body is made from the five elements and the five elements make up our unique constitution. We are all different in the balance of elements we have in the bodymind and in ayurveda these mixtures of elements are called doshas.

There are three specific doshas and we are all a combination of all three in varying amounts. These doshas are called vata, pitta and kapha. When everything is in balance we are in good health. Then we are said to be sattvic. However, as we know, life gets in the way and so we constantly find ourselves in varying states of imbalance. Things which can create an imbalance are foods, our daily routines, stress, climate, activity levels and type of activity plus where we choose to focus our attention in life. An imbalance occurs when we act in a way that causes one of the doshas, and the related elements, to increase or reduce and this then produces what we know as symptoms. These are all manifested physically as well as emotionally and psychologically. The descriptions below are brief but will give you a general idea.

At the end of this chapter you will find a dosha 'quiz'. You can use this to see what your dosha balance is like today. Remember that it changes all the time with daily life experiences, seasonal changes and the food we eat.

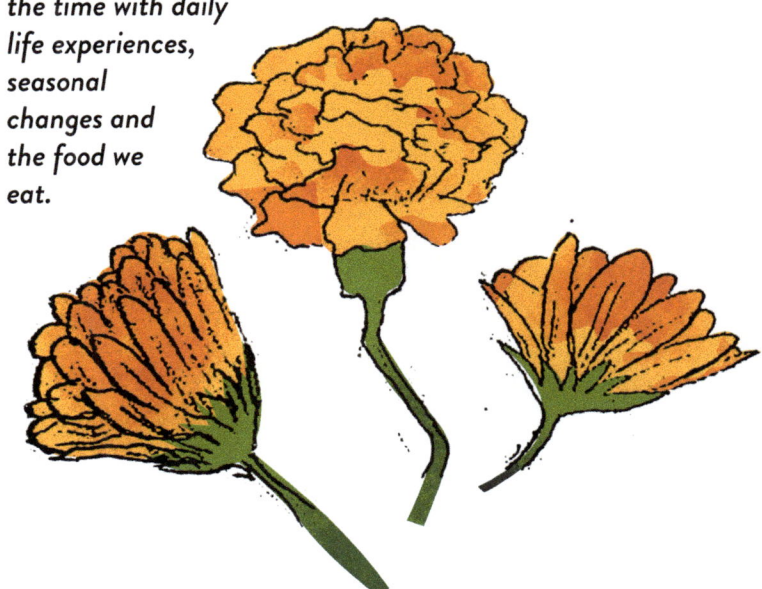

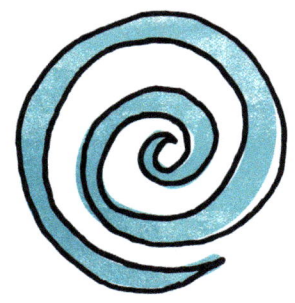

Vata comes from air and ether.

Vata qualities are light, dry, quick, cold.

Vata imbalance can manifest as IBS, constant change, insomnia, anxiety.

When in balance vata is physically flowing, creative, imaginative and vibrant.

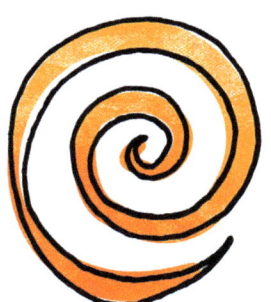

Pitta comes from fire and water.

Pitta qualities are hot, fiery and intense.

Pitta imbalance can manifest as inflammatory conditions, indigestion, skin inflammation, anger.

When in balance pitta is physically strong, organised, focused and intelligent.

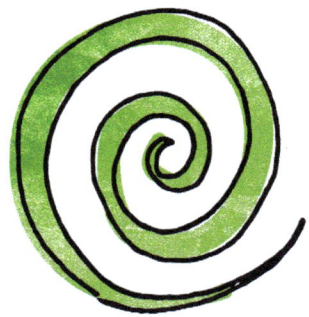

Kapha comes from water and earth

Kapha qualities are grounded, heavy, unctuous.

Kapha imbalance can manifest as excess mucus, especially to the chest and sinuses. It gets stuck physically as well as emotionally.

When in balance kapha is physically strong, grounded, loving and compassionate.

In addition to the different elements each dosha has a time of day where it is most prevalent. This then informs our recommended daily routine.

DOSHA	TIME OF DAY / NIGHT	WHAT TO CONSIDER
Vata (air and ether)	2am - 6am 2pm - 6pm	Vata is responsible for movement in the body. If you wake between 2am - 6am this is usually a sign that your Vata is imbalanced, there is too much movement. In the afternoon between 2pm - 6pm, if you have an energy dip, it's the same. You probably need to slow down.
Pitta (fire and water)	10am - 2pm 10pm - 2am	Pitta is responsible for transformation in the body. It is associated with our digestive fire, so turns food into energy. We should eat our main meal between 10am and 2pm because this is when Pitta, our digestion, is strongest. We need to be in bed resting by 10pm. Pitta governs the digestion at night with the liver and gall bladder. The body needs to be resting at this time for this to happen.
Kapha (earth and water)	6am - 10am 6pm - 10pm	Kapha is responsible for lubricating the body. It is advised that you get up around 7am. You are probably familiar with sleeping in late and feeling sluggish? This is because you have gone too far into the Kapha time. We naturally begin to feel tired in the evening. Eat a light supper by 7pm at the latest. Go to bed by 10pm. This is using this natural Kapha time to promote good sleep and rest.

The daily routine according to ayurvedic principles is in line with our circadian rhythms. Science has a lot to say about how how living in tune with these natural timings of day and night is hugely beneficial for our body and mind, and for our overall health and well-being.

DINACHARYA DAILY ROUTINE ESSENTIALS

Below is a list of everything you will need for a full daily self-care routine - dinacharya

Oil for mouth / oil pulling
(sesame or coconut culinary oil is fine)

Tongue scraper

Tooth brush /paste

Neti pot

Salt for neti, preferably nice himalayan variety

Body brush or good cloth

Body oil, dependent on your constitution
(grapeseed - kapha, coconut - pitta and almond - vata)

Nasaya oil

Lemon and hot water

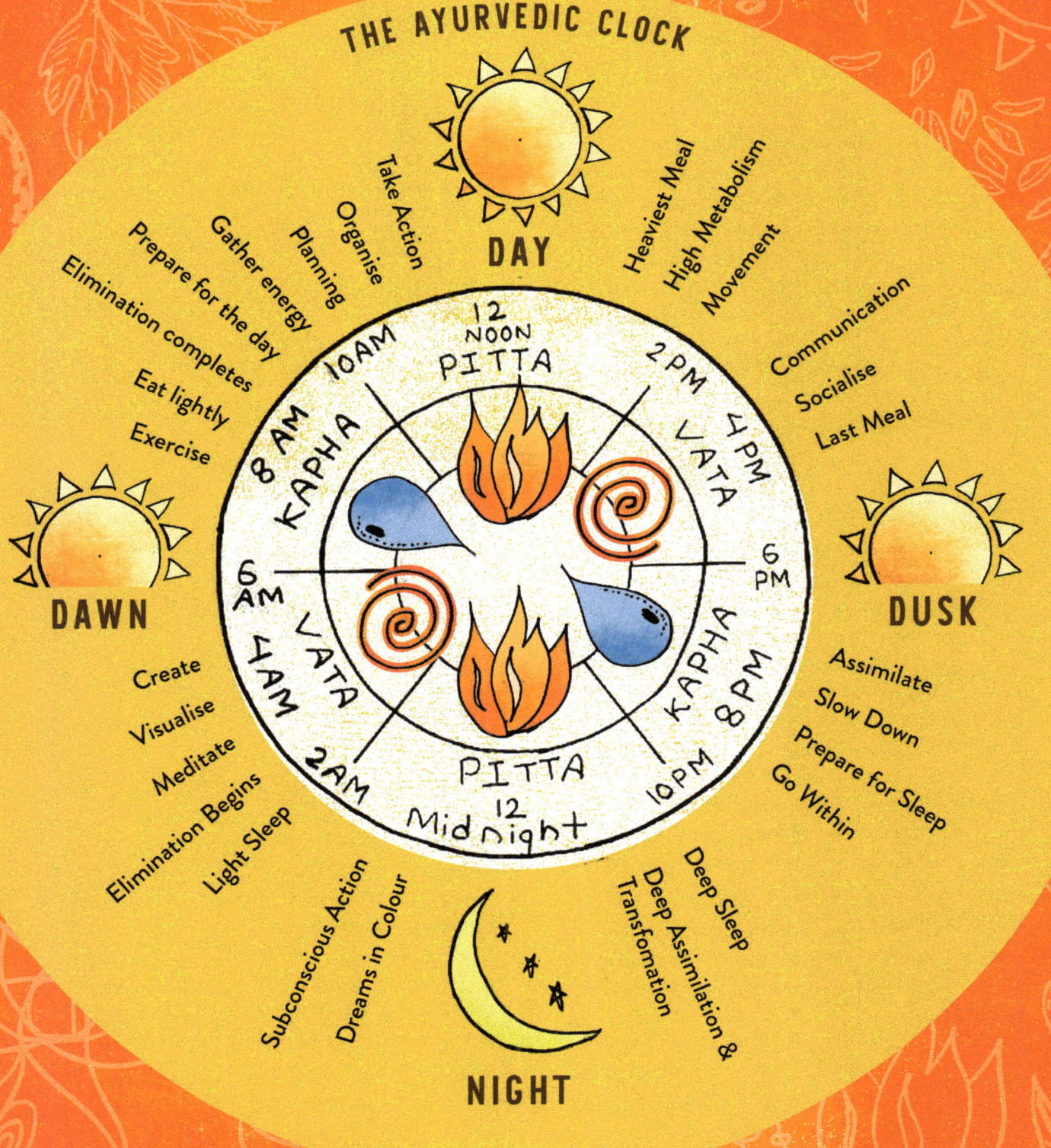

MORNING TIME.

It is suggested to rise between 6 - 8am. This is because if we stay in bed much after this we get a kind of sluggishness. You can see on the cyclical clock diagram that this is kapha time and so if we rest into the earthy grounded energy this begins the day with a heavy energy, we have taken on too much of the earth and water elements. This is also when our body naturally produces the hormone serotonin which wakes the bodymind up ready to begin the day. If we miss this peak we will not feel at our best and the whole body system will be affected and out of whack.

ROUTINE ON RISING.

It is a good idea to cleanse the body first thing in the morning, before eating or engaging with any daily tasks. Check out your tongue! It may have a coating on first thing in the morning. These are toxins in the body (ama). The following suggested morning routine can feel a little overwhelming at first so begin slowly with just one or two things, then when these begin to naturally feel part of what you do, introduce something else. Start with the thing you feel is most accessible for you. All of these practices have incredible benefits and are quite simple once you get going with them. Some of the techniques are best learned from a teacher who is experienced in them.

1. Oil pulling. Use sesame or coconut oil and put a good spoonful into your mouth and swill around for five minutes or so, like a mouth wash. Top tip: Spit the oil into the toilet afterwards so the sink doesn't get blocked).

2. Tongue scraping. You can use a spoon or a regular tongue scraper, to scrape all the residue off your tongue. Some people do this after the oil pulling some before, it's personal preference. Then brush your teeth.

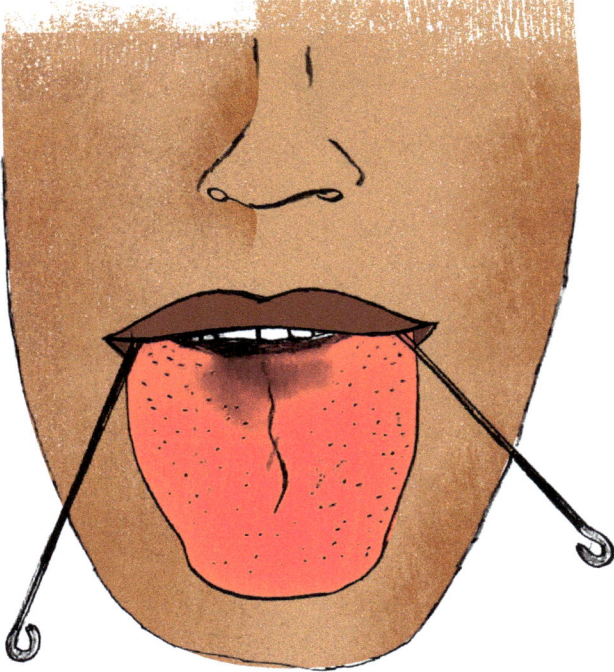

3. Cleansing breathing. This is my personal routine, I practice kapalbhati (rapid and vigorous) breathing each morning to fire up my system and get my metabolism going. If you are a less grounded person (more vata) or prone to heat (pitta) you may wish to do something a bit calmer. Either way the aim is to cleanse the nose for the next step. You may just prefer to give your nose a good blow. It is best to learn this breathing from an experienced teacher so you can check you're doing it correctly and also in a way that it is right for your constitution.

4. Neti. This is the practice of washing the nose and sinuses with warm salt water. Neti is done with a neti pot, a bit like a tiny watering can. It is extremely beneficial for respiratory health and for hay fever, infection and allergy prevention. The solution I use is one pinch of salt, use good quality salt for your body, in a cup full of warm body temperature water. It isn't essential to do this daily, but a couple of times a week is helpful. It's a good idea to ask someone experienced to go through it with you first.

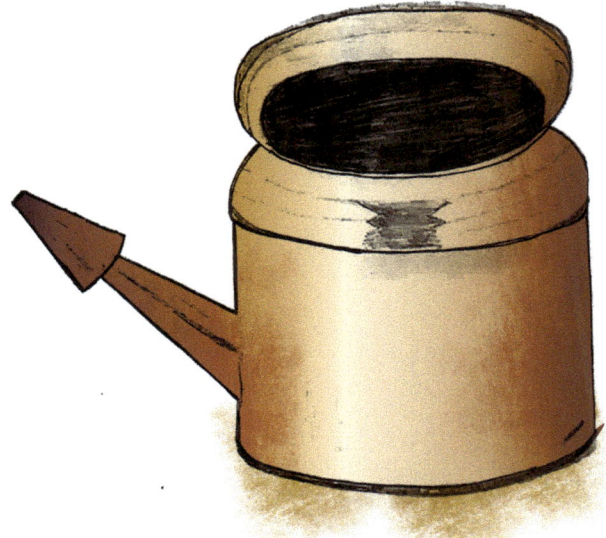

5. Nasaya oil. This oil is specifically for the nose. It is super helpful in preventing respiratory infections and allergic reactions and also helpful if you have dry nasal passages. There is also evidence that this practice, together with neti support the pituitary gland which is closely associated with your circadian rhythms, eating, sleeping and so on. Nasaya oil usually comes in a small bottle with a little pipette so you can squirt a small amount into each nostril after cleansing every morning.

6. Drink hot water with fresh lemon. This flushes and activates the digestive system. Please only do this after you have cleaned the mouth and nose as you want to avoid swallowing all the ama that is on your tongue.

7. Skin brushing. This is very beneficial in removing toxins that come out through the skin with sweat. You can get specific brushes, or use (gently) a loofah or a good cloth. Briskly 'brush' the limbs and then the torso in turn, brushing towards the heart. This practice improves circulation and helps detoxify the body. It is also helpful in reducing excess heat and congestion. It can help to disperse cellulite, is great for your skin, stimulates the lymphatic system and therefore helps with maintaining the body's immunity.

8. Oil your whole body. The name of this whole body oiling practice is abhyanga, this means love with oil. You can leave the oil on or alternatively shower or bath it off after 20 minutes. This is down to personal preference. This may sound time consuming but it can, once you get in to the routine, be done in 5 - 10 minutes. Different oils are recommended for different dosha types as follows:

Kapha, grapeseed oil (lighter as the skin can be oily and moist)

Pitta, coconut oil (cooling for easily irritated skin)

Vata, almond oil (nourishing for dry skin)

You can alternatively purchase specific oil for your unique constitutional type. Please see the recommended supplier section towards the end of this book for more details of where to purchase.

9. Do some kind of physical activity / exercise. This might be a walk, yoga, whatever works for you, but do move the body.

10. Meditation. Even if it is just five minutes sit quietly before properly beginning the day.

You will be pleased to hear that this is most of the dinacharya daily activities completed. The majority of the activity in this routine happens in the morning.

Abyangha – love with oil ♡

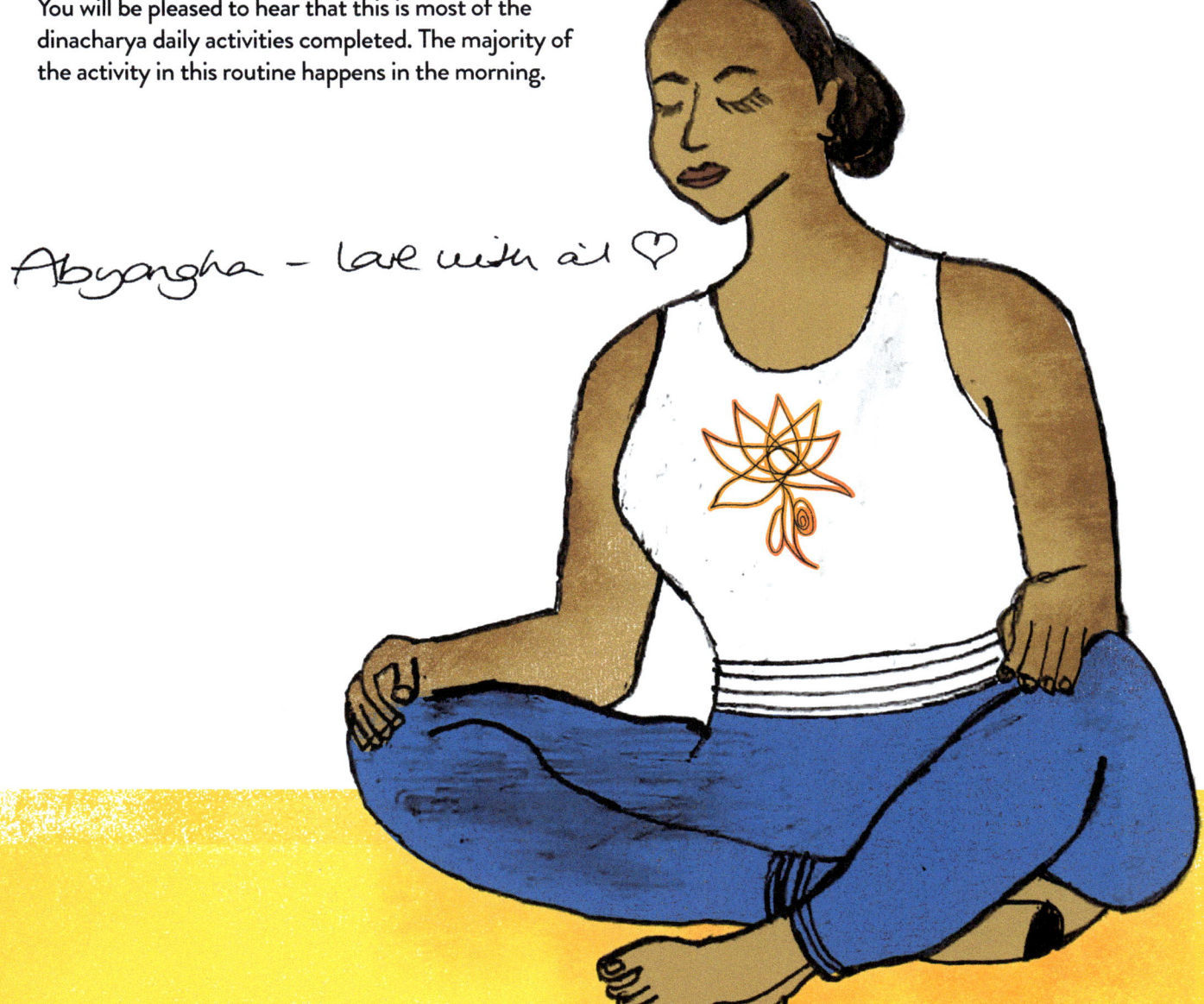

EATING.

The next consideration is mealtimes, which are suggested to coincide with when our digestion is working at its optimum. Our digestion is at its peak in the middle of the day when pitta dosha is the most dominant. So we ideally eat most of our food at this time.

Breakfast before 8:30am

Lunch between 12 - 2pm, the main meal of the day is eaten at lunch time

Supper before 7pm, this should be a light meal, soup or similar.

IT IS RECOMMENDED THAT MOST FOOD IS COOKED SO IT IS EASY FOR THE BODY TO DIGEST. NO RAW FOOD IN THE EVENINGS, AND FRUIT IS NOT MIXED WITH OTHER FOOD BECAUSE IT DIGESTS AT A DIFFERENT RATE, FERMENTS AND CAUSES DIGESTIVE ISSUES AND AMA (TOXINS). IN AYURVEDA DIGESTION IS OF THE UTMOST IMPORTANCE, ANY DISTURBANCE IN DIGESTION IS SEEN AS CREATING AMA WHICH CAN LEAD TO DIS-EASE.

SLEEPING.

Bedtime is by 10pm. This is in line with the circadian rhythm research. Our levels of melatonin hormone increase mid-evening and this is what helps us get off to sleep. If we miss this peak then we miss our sleep window and will most likely have a restless night. Sleep is vital for our health and healing.

ABOUT CIRCADIAN RHYTHMS.

Circadian rhythms ensure the body's functions are working appropriately at various points during a 24-hour period. Circadian rhythms exist in all types of living being including plants and animals, they even help flowers open and close at the right time.

In humans circadian rhythms coordinate mental and physical systems throughout the body. The digestive system produces proteins to match the typical timing of our meals. This rhythm is triggered by light and dark, day and night, which is why, if we are in balance, we naturally feel sleepy in the dark and if we have lots of artificial light and go against the rhythm, we can't sleep. The ayurvedic clock is aligned with this science.

HERE ARE SOME SLEEP WELL TIPS.

These tips are helpful for everyone but especially if you do have problems sleeping.

Avoid caffeine during the day. If you usually have difficulty sleeping, then avoid completely. If your sleep is ok then avoid caffeine after midday.

Avoid sugar in your food. This gives peaks and dips of energy which upset our rhythm in the body and disturbs sleep with cravings or energy surges.

Eat a light supper by 7pm at the latest. This should be soup or similar. No raw food. Nothing spicy or heating. This ensures the body is not still digesting food when you go to bed. If it is still digesting it will be difficult to settle and sleep and you may also feel overheated. In addition food may remain undigested and cause toxic build up in the body and digestive tract leading to gas, bloating, constipation and other digestive issues.

Have down time away from the computer or phone screens from 8pm. The pineal gland in the centre of the brain operates by increasing a hormone called melatonin which helps us to feel sleepy. If this is exposed to too much light it will believe it is still daytime and you won't feel sleepy. Switch devices off completely and read or listen to relaxing music.

Have a warm relaxing drink around 9pm, golden milk or a sleep tea (see pages 86 and 87).

Take care of your sleeping environment. If you find it relaxing have a bath and make the bedroom a welcoming and relaxing space, with nice lighting, oils and maybe a book to read. Make reading or anything else restful and not too stimulating, so no reading a horror story!

Go to bed by 10pm at the latest. This is essential for our body to repair itself. If we are not resting by this time then toxins will build up as the liver is not triggered to cleanse the body.

If you do wake in the night, or have trouble getting off to sleep, don't get up and start roaming about. Stay in bed and either listen to a relaxing yoga nidra or music. If you are familiar with breathing practices or meditation this can also be helpful.

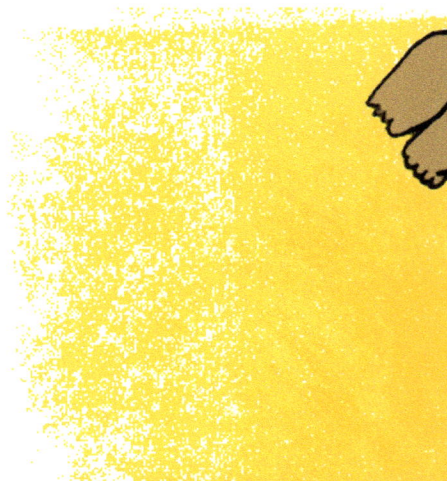

CIRCADIAN RHYTHMS EXIST IN ALL TYPES OF LIVING BEING INCLUDING PLANTS AND ANIMALS, THEY EVEN HELP FLOWERS OPEN AND CLOSE AT THE RIGHT TIME.

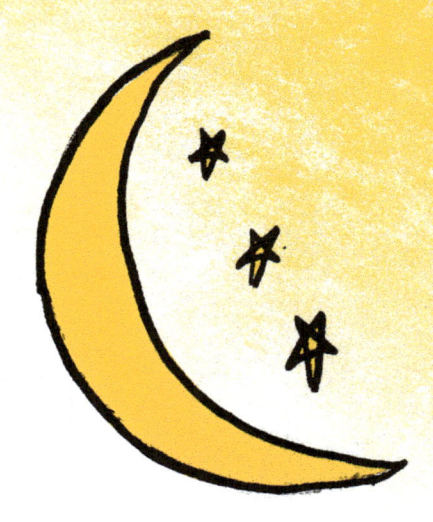
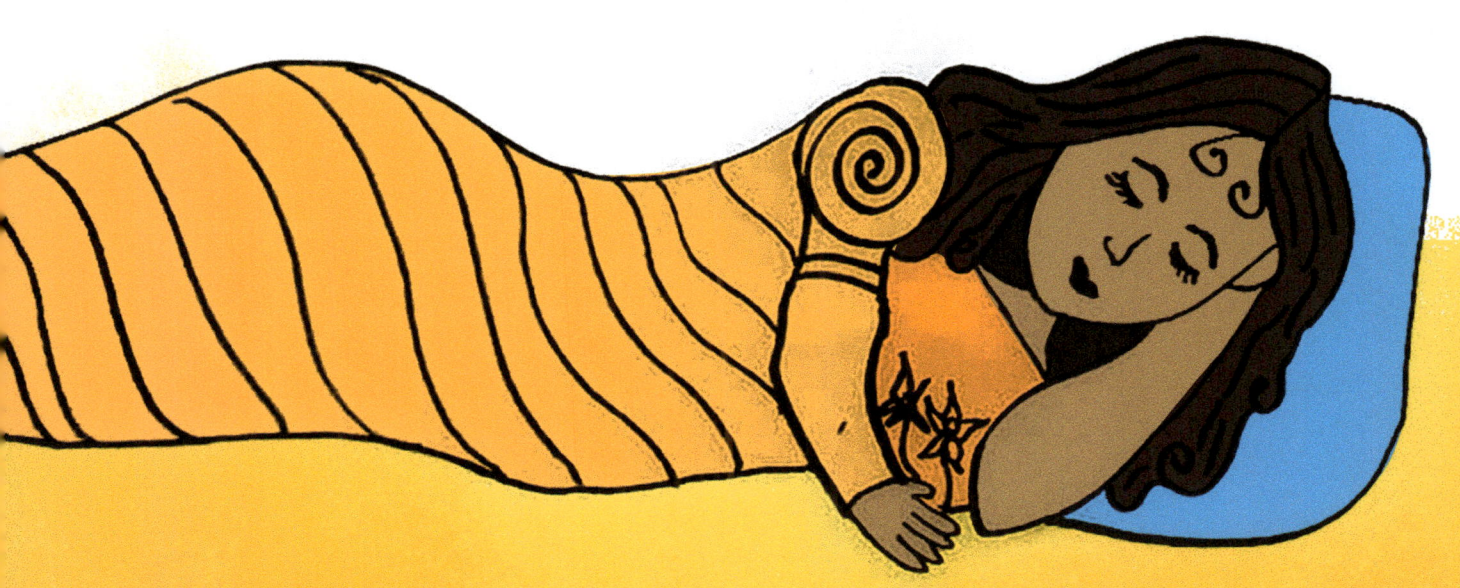

There are many food and lifestyle recommendations and practices for each dosha type. The following is a very brief summary.

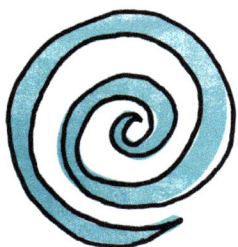

Vata increases with: Eating raw foods, salads, cold foods and dry foods like toast and crisps. Can be prone to having an erratic routine and can easily miss meals.

Calming for vata are: Regular meals, sweet grounding root vegetables, dairy and whole grains.

Vata can be too mobile so it is helpful for movement to be grounding and stabilising, walking in nature, yin or restorative yoga, for example.

Calming grounding breathing is great. Breath work is particularly helpful because air is the element of vata so we are directly calming the excess movement when we work with the breath.

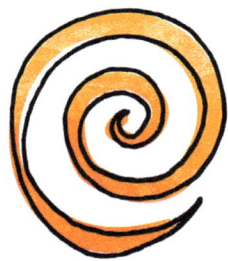

Pitta increases with: Too much heat, spicy hot foods, like chilli, lots of onion, caffeine, sugar, alcohol. Tends to struggle and feel angry if they miss meals.

Calming for pitta are: Leafy greens, sweet foods like root vegetables, creamy cooling things like coconut and yoghurt.

Pitta can be obsessive so benefits from moderate yet still challenging movement, and it is also helpful if it feels well structured. Cooling calming breathing is helpful for pitta as this cools the excess heat in the body and the hot temperament.

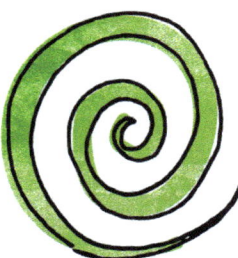

Kapha increases with: Dairy and other mucus forming foods such as tropical fruits, sugar, starchy and heavy foods. Can be prone to comfort eating.

Calming for kapha are: Lots of leafy greens, lighter foods, stimulating spices and not overeating.

Kapha can be sluggish so benefits from regular and fairly energetic movement. Cleansing and vigorous breathing is also helpful as the respiratory system can get congested.

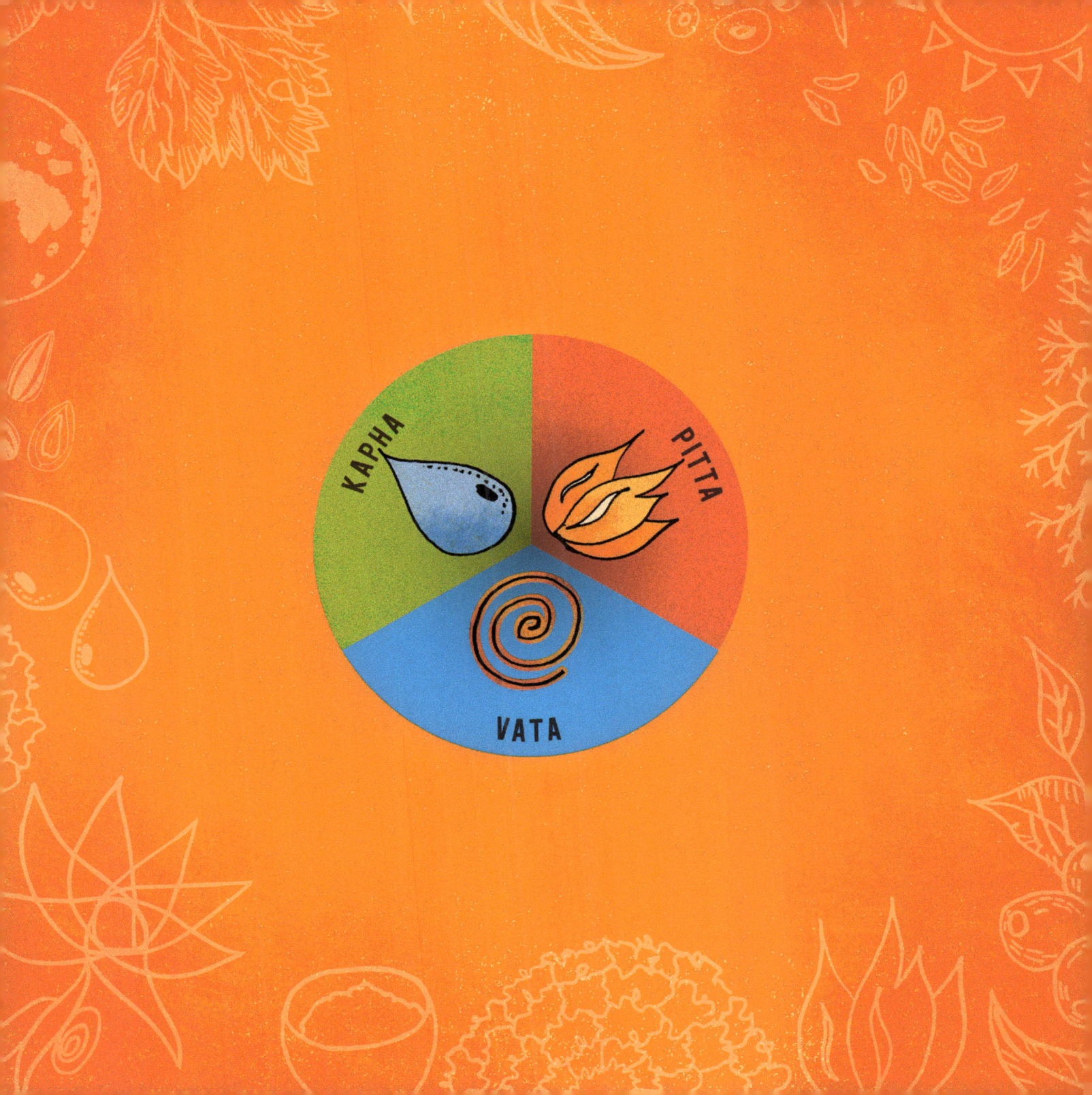

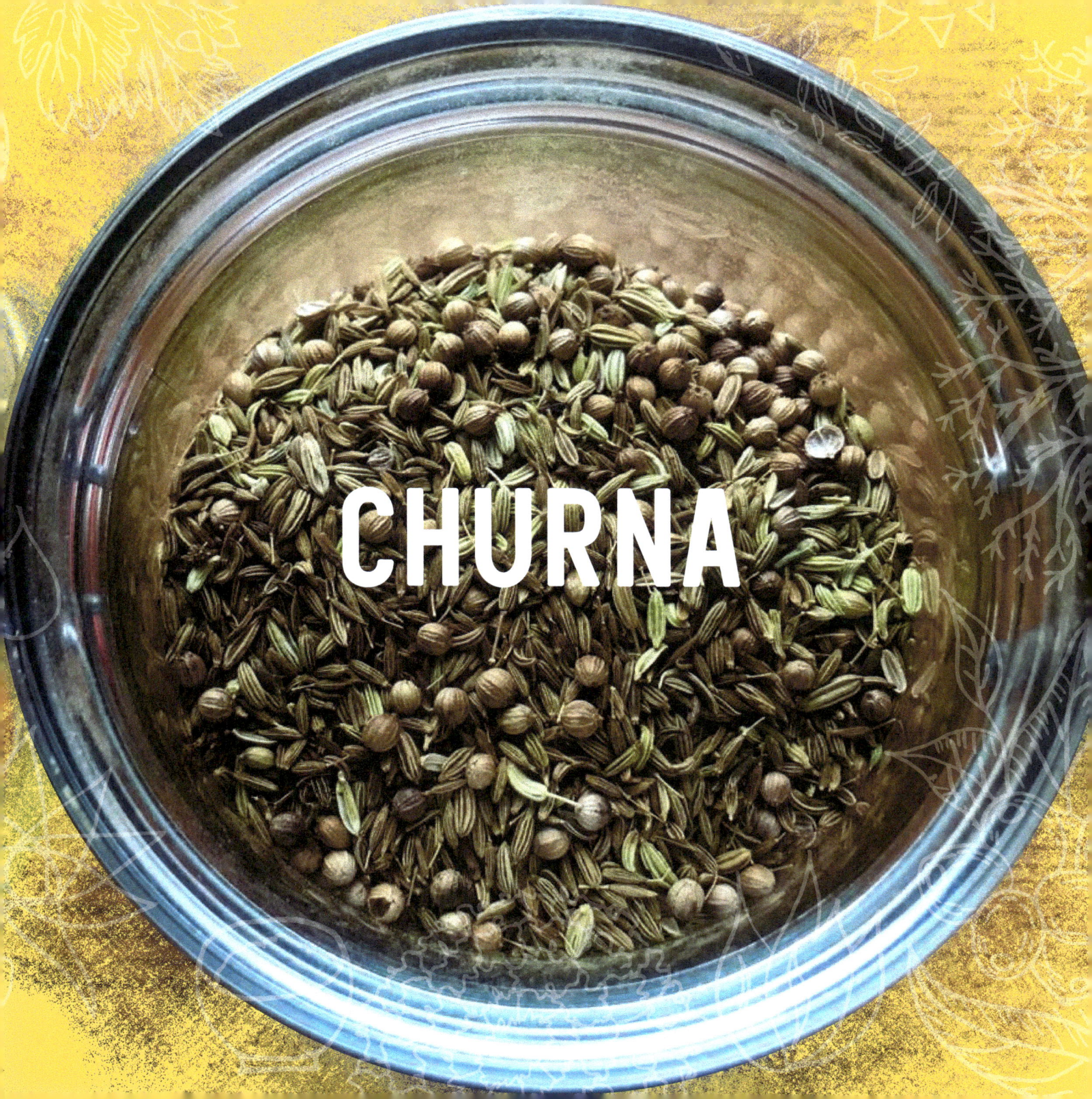

CHURNA RECIPES.

A churna is a mixture of spices and herbs that are helpful for balancing the constitution, and aiding digestion. They are delicious! They are simple to make. And they can be used with your food on a daily basis. They are also helpful if you are feeding several people with different constitutional needs as they can be sprinkled onto the food like a condiment before serving.

- Use daily with lunch and dinner.
- Use ½ to 1 teaspoon of the mix per meal.
- Measure the number of teaspoons listed for each of the ingredients and mix together.
- Store all the mixed spices in a jar or airtight container and keep in a cool place away from direct sunlight.
- You can toast the churna you are using in a dry pan before using each time.

A note on heat in the body: If you have excess heat in the body, please avoid the more fiery and heating spices. Excess heat may show up as feeling hot in your body, being hot tempered, hot skin rashes, indigestion or liver inflammation. Each recipe highlights where this may be the case.

KAPHA CHURNA.

8 teaspoons coriander seed

8 teaspoons cumin seed

6 teaspoons ground turmeric

Optionally (if you don't have heat issues in the body) add 2 teaspoons of ground ginger and 2 teaspoons of ground black pepper.

PITTA CHURNA.

10 teaspoons fennel seed

6 teaspoons coriander seed

6 teaspoons ground turmeric

VATA CHURNA.

8 teaspoons cumin seed

8 teaspoons fennel seed

2 teaspoons coriander seed

2 teaspoons ground turmeric

Optionally (if you don't have heat issues in the body) add 1 teaspoon of ground ginger and ¼ teaspoon of ground cinnamon.

A GUIDE TO YOUR AYURVEDIC CONSTITUTION.

Please note each section with the most relevant answer (V, P or K). Please take into account anything you are currently experiencing which is unusual or not your norm. If nothing quite fits please pick the closest answer. We all have all of the doshas (vata, pitta, kapha) within us in different quantities, there is no right or wrong response.

Add up all of your V, P, and K answers and note the total number for each in the bottom of each column. Sometimes two or all three are very similar. Sometimes one is obviously higher. And it changes throughout our life. This can then tell you if you are likely to be prone to any particular illness at the moment. For a more detailed analysis it is best to see a practitioner.

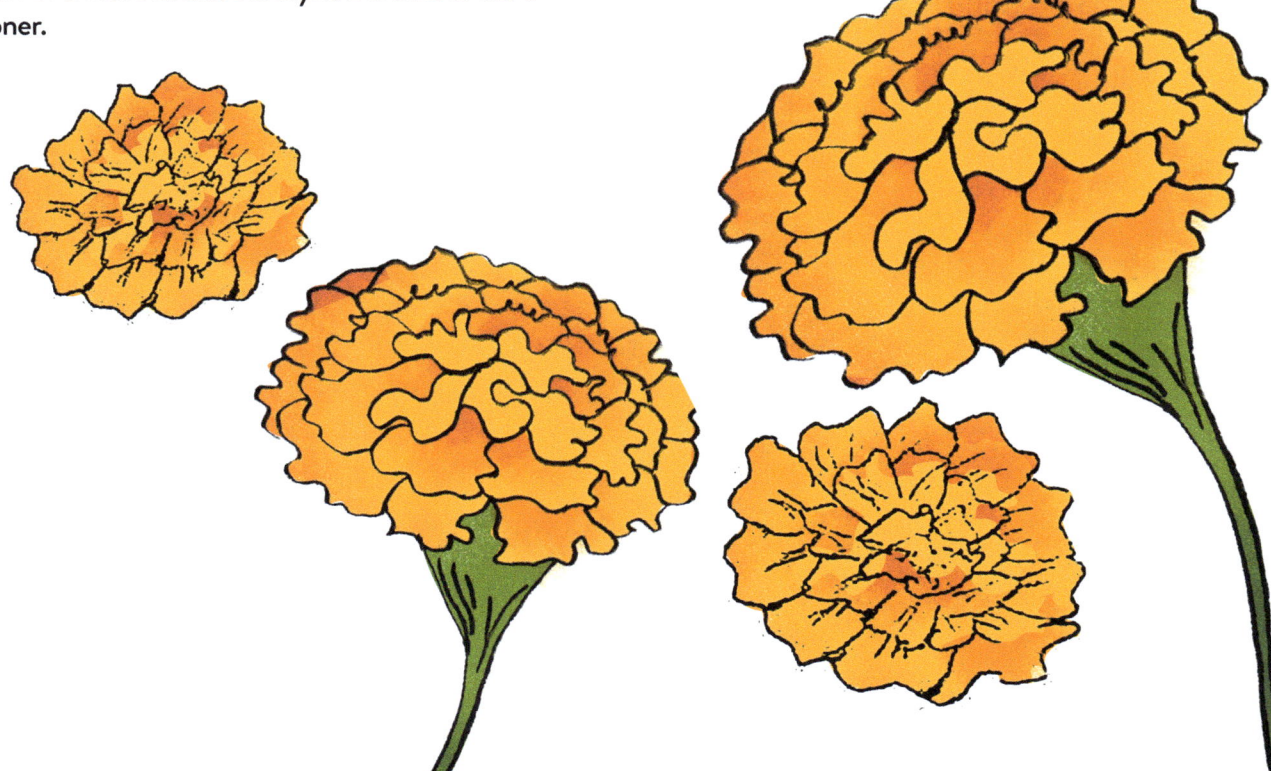

QUESTION	VATA	PITTA	KAPHA
YOUR BODY	Slim, bony	Medium, athletic, muscular	Larger frame
WEIGHT	Find it hard to gain weight	Fairly stable	Easy to gain weight
JOINTS	Cracking and clicking	Can be inflamed	Fluid retention
SKIN	Dry, scaly	Reddish and prone to inflammation	Oily, smooth
EYES	Small and beady	Intense and penetrating	Large and beautiful gaze
NOSE AND MOUTH	Dry nostrils no mucus	Can get inflammation maybe a sore throat, mouth ulcers	Mucous and blocked nose and sinuses
TONGUE	Dry and cracked	Inflamed, yellow coating	Pale, white coating
HAIR	Thin and dry	Early greying, oily	Thick and luscious
BODY TEMPERATURE	Cold, especially hands and feet	Warm, sometimes too hot	Warm, but cold if damp
ILLNESS YOU ARE USUALLY PRONE TO	IBS, constipation, anxiety	Ulcers, skin rashes, inflammation	Chest infections, sinusitis.
APPETITE AND DIGESTION	Easily misses meals	Good appetite, doesn't like to miss meals	Enjoys food, can overeat
SLEEP	Poor, wakes often	Adequate	Can sleep a lot
TEMPERAMENT	Lively, imaginative	Focused, determined	Loving, compassionate
REACTION IF STRESSED	Anxious	Angry	Withdrawn
TOTAL			

GET IN TUNE WITH THE MOON

Lunar beauty
shines upon us.
Ever changing,
energy rising
and falling away.
Cyclical shifting
move with it
become her.

WHAT IS CYCLICAL WISDOM?

It is the cycles of life, of our lives on this earth and of life in its wider sense. From heatwaves to the ice age, day to night, seasons and the earth moving around the sun, everything is constantly shifting and changing in a cyclical pattern.

Energy is not linear. Everything that is a living or earthly entity has an energy within it. I believe this energy pattern to be a kind of spiral or circling type force, which is why things often repeat or return to where they began, or very similar, and why things seem so cyclical. There are many of these different cycles that we can see in nature.

The seasons of the year in some parts of the world and different climates provide a definitive example of shifting and changing. We can view the summertime or hottest season, with the energy from the sun and longer days filled with light, as being akin to the full moon with the energy at its height. As the heat slowly dissipates into cooler weather this is much more like the slowly waning moon. Inevitably autumn always brings us to winter, which can be soft, still and quiet, much like the new moon, dark and silent. And the newness which comes right after the new moon with its waxing energy is like the energy of springtime, with a promise of vibrancy and newness everywhere.

These energetic changes can also be tangibly experienced with the human breath cycle. The breath is our link to the unconscious mind and emotions, it is something we can allow to be passive or we can use it to help ourselves feel differently, to shift our emotional state. The pause at the end of the in-breath is where we have the most energy held in the body, summertime. This is also our habit if we feel uptight or anxious, to hold the breath in. As we breathe out there is an instinctive and intuitive letting go, the autumn time of the breath cycle, a release. In the pause at the end of the out-breath is that perfect stillness of winter. As we breathe in again we welcome new energy in to the bodymind, this is similar in our Western seasons to springtime energy.

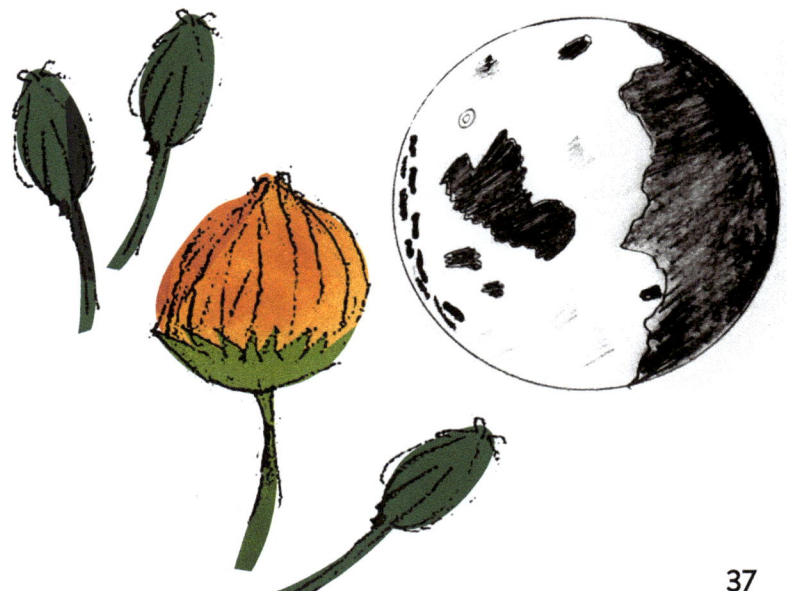

The moon cycles, seasons and breath cycles can all be transposed onto the ayurvedic model of the three gunas. These gunas are three differing energies that constantly shift and change. The gunas are present in everything in nature and are also used to describe and understand our state of mind.

Tamas: This is a dull, inert and stuck, heavy and lazy or low mood kind of energy. Tamas, with its dullness would be more aligned with the new moon and its quietness.

Rajas: This is an overexcited, high, restless and agitated energy state. Rajas is more in harmony with the full moon with this energy at its height.

Sattva: This is the third guna that describes what is it to be sattvic. This is a state of perfect equilibrium, physically, psychologically and spiritually.

(For more information on gunas see page 49).

THE THIRD GUNA IS SATTVA, OR BEING SATTVIC. THIS IS A STATE OF PERFECT EQUILIBRIUM, PHYSICALLY, PSYCHOLOGICALLY AND SPIRITUALLY.

We can understand all of these energetic states in terms of our human experience. Women in particular have a definitive and tangible cyclical experience through their lives. The process of menstruating is in and of itself an amazing cyclical experience.

We are all different, however it is fairly common to ovulate at the full moon when the energy is at its height, and to menstruate on the new moon which then naturally with the winter stillness and darkness becomes a time to rest. After we no longer bleed, or if we have never bled regularly, the moon cycle can be a wonderful guide and we can use this to consistently follow some cyclical awareness in our day to day life. This teaches us that sometimes we need to rest, and at other times we feel more energetic. We constantly shift and change, our energy constantly ebbs and flows.

These energetic patterns that we can become so familiar with can also include the elements and the doshas, which are our constitutional states in ayurveda. These elements and doshas are also a part of the female cycle. As the restful new moon energy leaves us the spring energy in our systems increases. We leave the grounded (kapha dosha) earth energy and begin to become more fiery. This fiery feeling (pitta dosha) builds even more after we have ovulated, or experienced the full moon, and continues to build with the fire energy still growing. The intensity of the building fire creates a movement and restlessness associated with the air and ether elements, (vata dosha), where we may menstruate, until the new moon when we may again feel more restful and return to the earth. These different energies of the ayurvedic doshas all have different seasonal representations, but also times of day (as in the ayurvedic clock on page 23), because within each climate are individual days and each day is also cyclical.

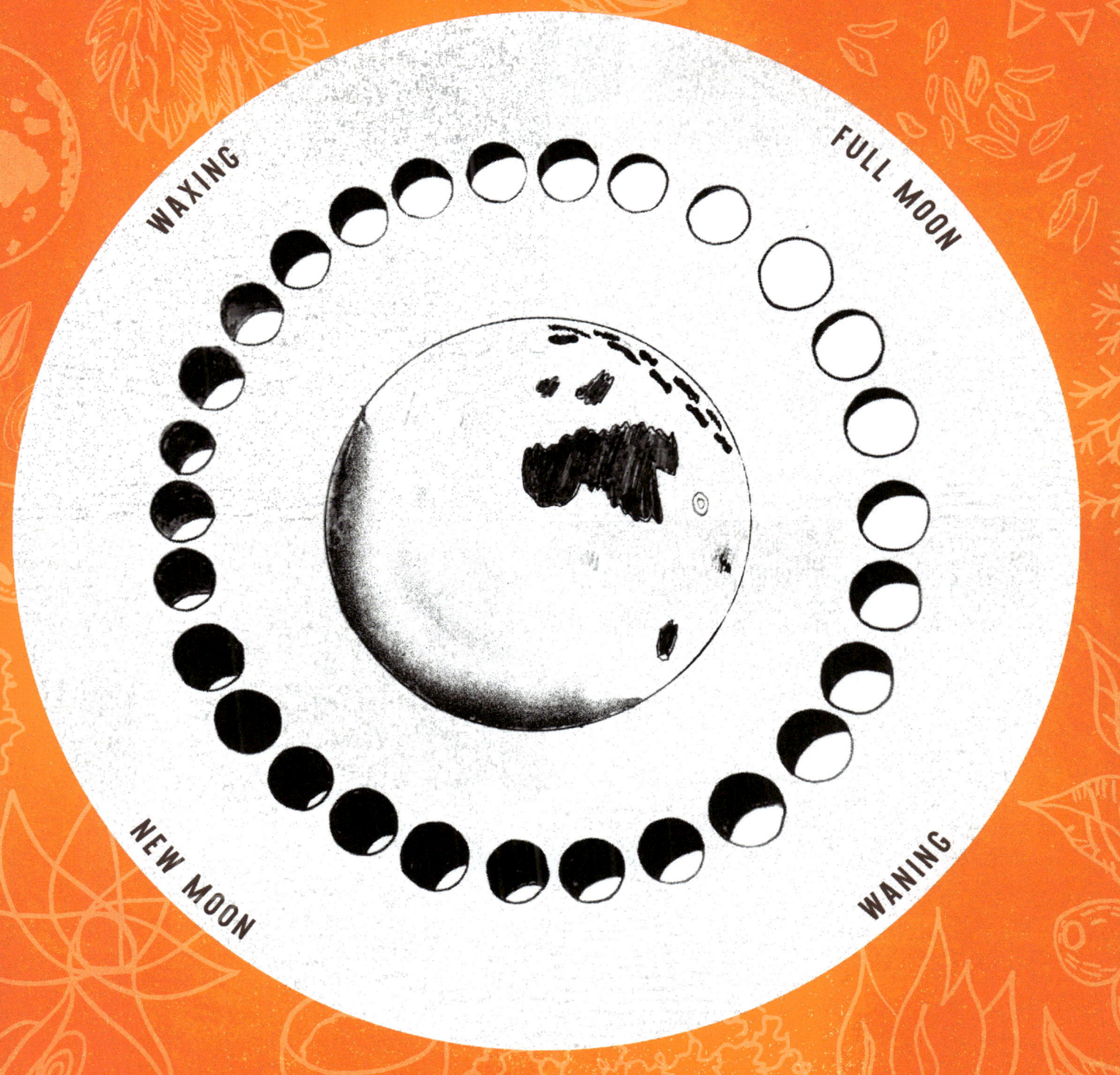

If we can have a basic understanding of these shifting and fluid energies in life, and within ourselves, we can begin to use them to our advantage. We can begin to work with them to obtain and maintain our health and wellness, on a physical, psychological and emotional level.

All of what I am sharing with you is aimed at promoting an understanding of all of these energies and their qualities. I know from personal experience that we can be completely responsible for our own health and well-being. We can feel within the digestive system of the body the difference between eating a pizza or some fresh vegetables. We can make time to notice the seasons as they change. Learn to rest when we need to. We can choose to make time for self-care practices in our daily life and to prioritise our own health and wellness. So often in this busy world we ignore the changing and shifting seasons, lunar cycles, times of day. We push, push, push until we are exhausted. And then we still push some more. We ignore this precious and incredible cyclical wisdom that we are gifted as part of our being human. We forget that we are part of nature's wisdom. We overwork, overdo and then collapse, exhausted. Only then may we finally begin to listen. Only then may we begin to become human beings instead of human doings.

THE MOON.

In ayurveda and yoga texts and systems the moon is a feminine force. Watery, ebbing and flowing, ever changing, gentle and nurturing. The moon is the ultimate cycle. She is literally above and beyond us. Hanging in the sky the moon is not controlled or coerced by the human race, and we are somewhat beholden to her influence over us. As the visibility of the moon waxes and wanes so do the tides, and so do our emotional states.

At full moon the energy is at its height, hence the term lunatic. It is well known in healthcare services such as emergency departments that frantic activity and bizarre behaviour is markedly increased at this phase of the moon. Therefore the energy of the full moon can be observed to affect how we are feeling. Amazingly the fluid known as interstitial fluid within the human body is exactly the same chemical composition as seawater. This fluid is found in the interstitial spaces, the tissue spaces in between all of the cells. On average a human has about eleven litres of interstitial fluid that provide the cells with nutrients and as a means of waste removal. It should therefore be no surprise that the moon affects us, as she certainly affects the water within the earth's oceans.

We can use the energy of the moon psychologically as well as noticing how it may affect our bodily rhythms. If the full moon is the height of energy then the new moon can be viewed as a time to rest and restore, a more quiet 'dark moon' time. It is kind of like switching the lights on and off. When it's dark we rest. When it's light we are naturally more active. Traditionally the full moon is the peak, after which you can let things go, as the moon slowly reduces in visibility. When the moon has reached her full peak and begins to wane, this is an excellent time for focusing on letting go of anything you no longer need. The dark new moon is the new beginning. Emerging from the darkness into a time of focusing and manifesting change, with the moon gradually increasing in visible size and energetic influence. We can set intentions after the new moon, the idea is that the energy of the intentions grow with the moon energy.

Full moon letting go
New moon manifest

RITUALS.

A ritual is simply a particular routine that has meaning for you. In the context of this book it would be something that is personal to you, that will help you to focus and bring about whatever you need for nurture and self-care. There are so many ways of approaching this and you really can make it your own. There are not any specific rules unless you wish to follow a particular tradition, then you may need to research a bit more. You can include (or not) any objects, photographs, plants or anything else that means something to you and maybe has significance for your intent with the ritual. It's also nice to have a candle or two and if you like some incense or essential oils. If you want to sing, play an instrument, write, chant or talk out loud you can do that too.

As a helpful suggestion, I was taught from a Buddhist school that you can include the following things (this is not essential but a nice guideline): Flowers (impermanence), incense (cleansing and purification of the space), light (a candle, for the eyes to focus upon), perfume (sense of smell), a little bell (sound and hearing). I also use a little bowl of rice, sometimes people use water. These things are all made as an offering to whatever energy or entity you are directing the ritual towards. So in this case it may be the moon, or it may be associated with your intention.

SETTING AN INTENTION.

Within these rituals there is the suggestion to set an intention or a focus. This is ideally not something you think about with the mind but something more instinctive and intuitive. It is also not something to pressure yourself into doing. The following may be helpful guidance for intention setting.

When walking in nature or sitting quietly alone notice anything that comes into your thoughts. Dreams, hopes, desires and fears. Especially notice anything that keeps arising again and again.

Write things down, thoughts, feelings, desires. Try not to make this goal driven, it is deeply personal and led not from the head but from the heart. Create, if you feel like it. Draw, write, paint, dance, sing, do whatever you feel. Express yourself. In this self-expression we allow the agenda placed upon us to drop away and we reconnect with our real sense of what is important for us in this world. Keep it positive. Focus on what life will be like once this has come into being. Let go of negativity and of what you no longer need and focus on what you wish for more of.

Your intention doesn't need to be in words, it can be a feeling, an emotion, a visualisation. It is yours, do it however you feel resonates with you. An intention can be something very simple, for example wishing yourself love, peace and happiness.

Particularly when focusing on letting go it is important to do this with love and compassion, kindness towards whoever or whatever you wish to release. When welcoming in something new don't be greedy! Do this with gentle awareness, no expectations, but a belief that it can happen.

MOON BATHING.

A beautiful practice is that of moon bathing. This can be bathing as you would in the sun but in moonlight instead, outdoors in nature, or indulging in a herbal bath. If you don't have a full-size bath you can use a bowl and do this as a foot bath instead. It's important to note that when using herbs in a bath we absorb the potency of these mixtures through the skin, so do be aware of the stated contraindications and be cautious if necessary. You don't need to avoid the bath altogether, just leave out that particular herb.

FULL MOON RITUAL.

Take time to find a quiet outside space, aim for this to be somewhere where what you are going to leave out won't be eaten or meddled with by passing wildlife (I speak from experience!). Place an apple and a glass of water outside under the light of the full moon. You may wish to add to this by using a cloth and creating a kind of alter. For example, crystals are said to be cleansed of negative energy and charged in the full moon light, plus you can add any other sacred objects you feel. As you set things out take time to consider anything you may wish to let go of following this full moon night. Sit for a while and gaze at your ritual objects and at the moon, then go inside for a herbal bath.

The following morning rise early at dawn and go to collect your apple and water. Sit in your peaceful outside space with your objects that have now been bathed and blessed by the moon herself. Eat the apple mindfully and drink the water. Feel you are now ingesting and embodying the qualities of the female force of the full moon and of whatever intention you set as you focused on them the previous evening.

FULL MOON BATH.

Prepare the bathroom space with candles, ensure it's warm and cosy and that you have everything to hand, bath herb decoction (see below), anything you wish for your ritual, any oil, pyjamas for after your bath.

1 tablespoon dried calendula
1 tablespoon dried rose
1 tablespoon dried lemon balm
1 cup epsom salts (optional)

1. Put the herbs into a pan and fill with water (about a litre is enough).

2. Simmer for 15 minutes with a lid on then strain through a sieve into a hot bath.

3. Add epsom salts to the bath if you wish

Calendula is anti-inflammatory, calming for the musculoskeletal system, can ease menstruation cramps and is antibacterial.
Not recommended during pregnancy.

Rose is healing for the heart. Cooling for a fiery temperament, healing for the skin, calming and soothing for the mood and emotions.

Lemon balm is incredibly helpful for calming the nervous system, reliving anxiety and easing exhaustion. It eases low moods and is said to lighten the heart. It is also said to help with concentration. Lemon balm is considered very supportive for meditation as it brings balance to the heart and mind.
Avoid with barbiturates for insomnia or anxiety as it may increase their effects.

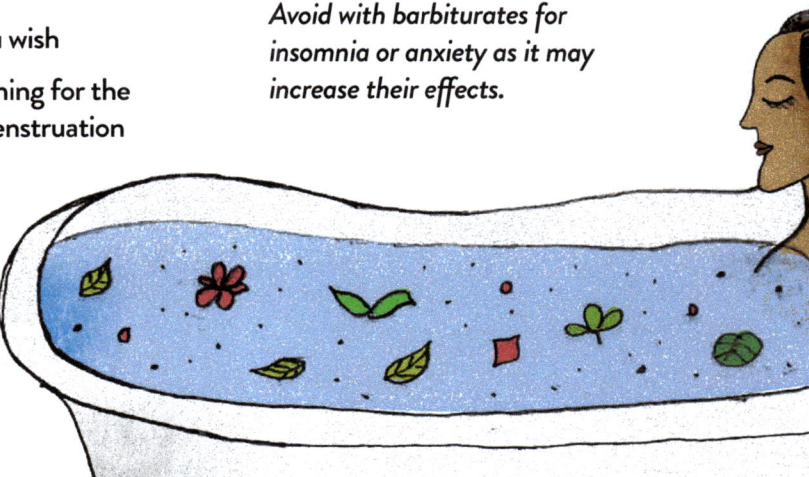

NEW MOON RITUAL.

I begin preparing things a few days before the new moon - this isn't essential but I have found it very helpful. The time as we approach the new moon is the most powerful time for letting go, which we began with the full moon ritual. For at least one day just before the new moon consider doing a simple dietary cleanse. I do this on whatever day fits best in my schedule so it can alter slightly. If you have the time and the inclination maybe even do this for three days or more. This can incorporate just the dietary aspects, maybe also taking some castor oil to enhance the effect and perhaps a herbal enema (please seek support from a practitioner if you wish to learn to do this). The castor oil really enhances the gut and full body cleansing. Old food that is stuck in the digestive system is softened and then moved out of the body as a result. This stuck waste can eventually create toxins which then lead to disease so this is an excellent preventative practice and is especially enhanced by the letting go process that naturally occurs with the new moon. This fully cleanses the colon where we can hold onto so much emotionally and energetically (for more detailed information on cleansing see page 99).

The focus as the new moon arrives is on shedding that which we no longer need, and then on resting for a while, before bringing in the new. This is a time of complete darkness, from which anything we desire can arise. Think of it as a seed buried in the dark soil, waiting to burst forth into the light.

Prepare a simple space, with any crystals or appropriate objects of your choosing, be inside this time in the warm and with candles to celebrate the soon to return light. Know that after darkness the light always returns. Focus on the light of a flickering candle. Allow the light to permeate you, feel as though you are absorbing this fully, through your skin deep into your physical being, light filling your tissues cells and organs. Allow your mind to feel filled with light, and feel you are made of light. Now gently close the eyes and imagine this same light illuminating your heart centre, beneath your breastbone in the centre of the chest. Sit with this for as long as you feel comfortable.

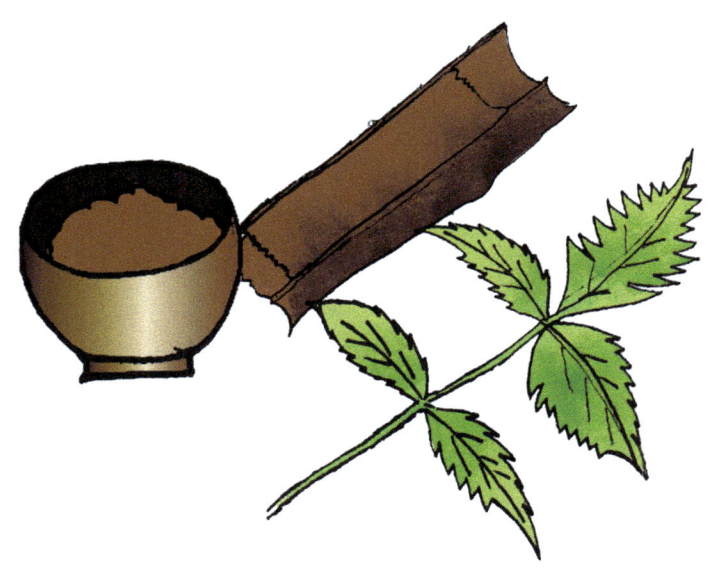

NEW MOON BATH.

1 tablespoon dried camomile
1 tablespoon dried lavender
1 tablespoon dried skullcap
1 tablespoon dried tulsi
1 cup epsom salts (optional)

1. Put the herbs into a pan and fill with water (about a litre is enough).

2. Simmer for 15 minutes with a lid on then strain through a sieve into a hot bath.

3. Add epsom salts to the bath if you wish

Camomile relieves insomnia, eases anxiety, calms digestion and soothes irritated skin. *Not to be taken during pregnancy or breastfeeding or if you have a bleeding disorder.*

Lavender improves mood, promotes restful sleep, relieves stress and reduces inflammation

Skullcap boosts mood, reduces anxiety, is antibacterial and antiviral, anti-inflammatory, soothes the nervous system and relieves insomnia. *Do not take alongside other tranquilizers or sedatives.*

Tulsi relieves stress and anxiety, is antibacterial and antiviral, anti-inflammatory and is good for respiratory health. Tulsi is considered a sacred medicinal plant in India. *May thin the blood so avoid if on anticoagulant medicines, avoid in pregnancy and breastfeeding.*

Following these baths you may wish to oil your body, to lie and rest or to enjoy some meditation or yoga nidra. Depending on the time of day you may also wish to have a light supper. Keep everything very quiet and mindful. These herbal bath decoctions are incredibly powerful and it is best to rest afterwards.

IN A WORLD WHERE WE CAN GET SO EASILY CAUGHT UP IN THE EXTERNAL AGENDA OF SOCIETY. TUNING INTO NATURE'S RHYTHM IN THIS WAY IS COMFORTING AND CALMING. IT GIVES US AN INTERNAL SENSE OF REASSURANCE. IT OFFERS A RHYTHM TO OUR DAYS AND A FOCUS TO OUR BODYMIND. IT CREATES A SENSE OF EQUILIBRIUM AND EQUANIMITY. IT SHOWS US HOW TO SELF-CARE AND SELF-LOVE. HOW TO LIVE IN TUNE WITH NATURE. IT IS SIMPLE, YET POWERFUL. IT IS HOW WE ALWAYS USED TO BE AND SO IT RECONNECTS US WITH OURSELVES.

BECOMING SATTVIC

Hot and cold
light and dark
fire and ice
heavy and light
contrasting and comparing
opposites attract
then fade away
into sattva.

These are three gunas:

1. Rajas is light, high energy, fast and hot
2. Tamas is dark, inert, slow and cool
3. Sattvic is balanced, light, joyous, balanced and pure

WHAT DOES BECOMING SATTVIC ACTUALLY MEAN?

Being sattvic is a state of equanimity, health and happiness with balance in the bodymind. To become sattvic we go through a process, of shedding anything which disturbs this balance, a process of letting go. To become sattvic we change our routine, food, lifestyle, habits. We embrace practices that help us feel more at peace and in tune with ourselves and the rhythms and cycles of nature. We come back to ourselves as we truly are. As we gradually shift and change our habits we find we naturally begin to feel more balanced, less agitated or restless. We are then beginning to experience becoming sattvic.

Life is a constant interplay of elemental energy, as we have seen in the previous chapters with the elements, moon cycles and the doshas. Within this system we also have another kind of energy and this is the gunas.

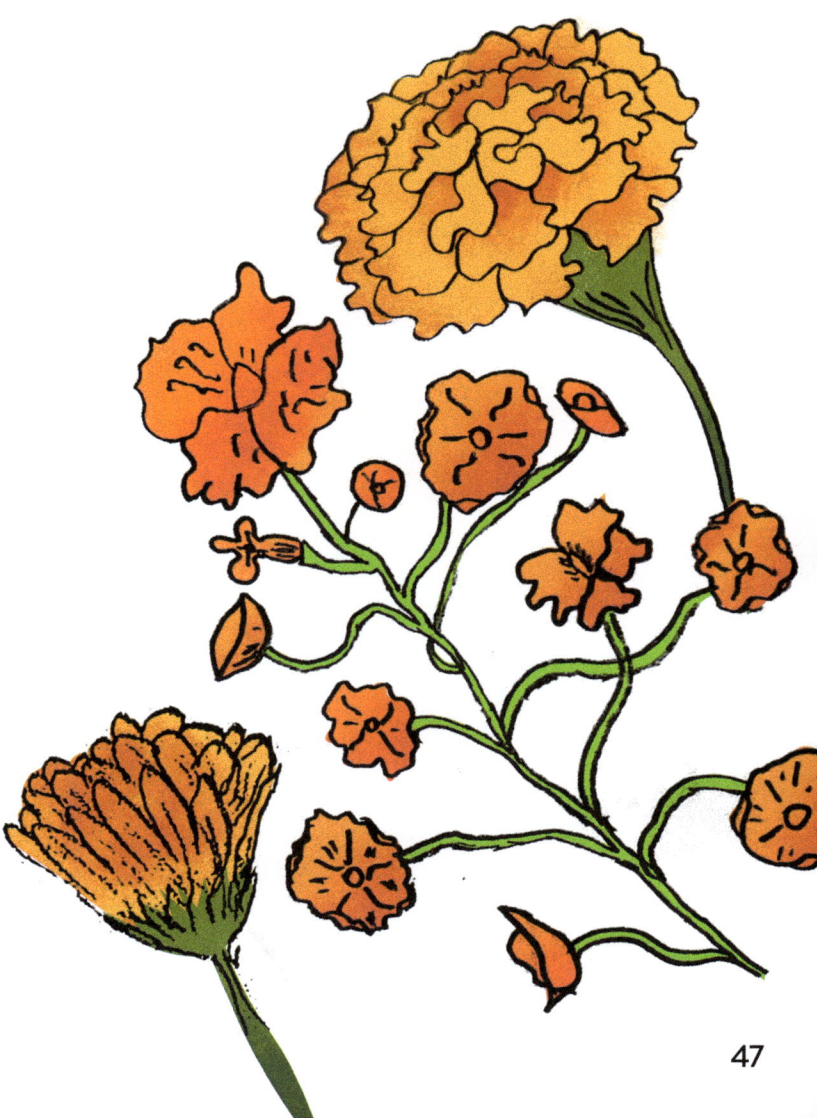

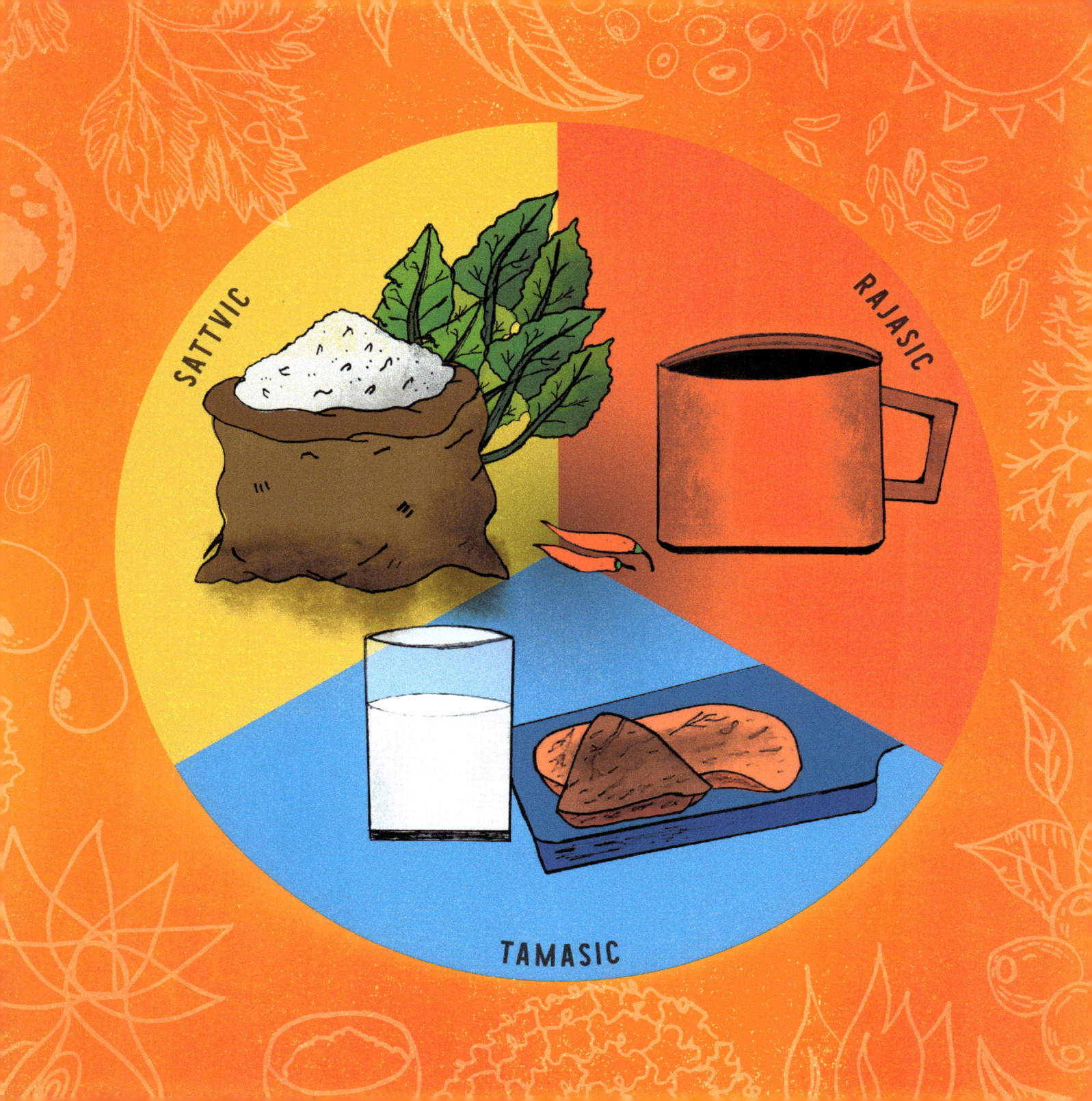

THE GUNAS.

The gunas are energetic states that are found within everything - in plants, animals, foods, the environment and the seasons. For example a cold dark and damp winter day is more of a tamasic state, whilst a hot mid-summer day with sunshine is rajasic. These energies and qualities can affect our own energetic (dosha) balance. We can see how on a damp winter day we are more likely to feel sluggish and like staying indoors, less active. Whilst in sunny warm weather we may feel more naturally inclined to be outdoors and active. The gunas are also sometimes used to describe our mental health or state of mind.

We can bring this energetic awareness into our everyday life to help ourselves to feel more balanced and sattvic.

THE SATTVIC STATE IS LIGHT YET GROUNDED, JOYOUS YET EVEN TEMPERED, HEALTHY AND HAPPY YET REALISTIC. THERE IS COMPLETE CLARITY OF THOUGHT AND ACTION AS WELL AS A SENSE OF INNER KNOWING AND DEEP PEACE.

By balancing our energies, physical, psychological and emotional, we may begin to experience this more sattvic state.

If activities, climate or our environment, including other people around us, are more rajasic in nature this may affect and impact upon how we feel. We could become more rajasic ourselves, or perhaps become exhausted and more tamasic. Equally if we are in a more tamasic environment or around people who are less active we may have a tendency to be more like this too. If we adopt one or other of these states or both at various times this can create dis-ease.

An excess of rajas can cause eventual exhaustion, if we continuously operate at high speed, excess energy and a constant hyper vigilant state we will exhaust ourselves in the end. If we are tamasic then we are not active enough and things become stagnant and stuck, this creates physical and psychological blockages in the bodymind. Psychologically we can see rajas and tamas in extremes in a bi-polar diagnosis for example, we find tamas in depression and rajas in hypermanic states.

To some extent we all fluctuate between rajas and tamas most of the time. This is human nature, what we ideally strive for is a sense of sattvic balance. The soul is said to always be sattvic, it's just that life gets in the way and we don't have the time or space to notice this place of inner peace.

To calm rajas we need to slow down, walk in nature, practice grounding yoga, slow breathing and meditation. To lift ourselves up from tamas we need to walk outdoors, get more active, practice energising yoga, stimulating breathing and walking meditation. We can learn to balance these states with our daily routine, cyclical awareness, herbs, massage, yoga, breathwork and the food we eat.

Foods are also rajasic, tamasic or sattvic. This book is of course called Sattvic Soul. Most of the recipes I am sharing with you are therefore sattvic. This means they are good for most people, will help you to feel satisfied and well-fed, not overly full, nicely energised and beautifully nourished.

BALANCING THINGS OUT WITH FOOD.

In case you're feeling sluggish or hyper it's useful to know what may help. Then you can adjust your diet accordingly and this will usually even things out. Rajasic foods include caffeine (coffee and chocolate), alcohol, refined sugar, wheat. Tamasic foods include meat and fish, dairy (cheese, milk, yoghurt), refined sugar, wheat and alcohol. I am not saying do not ever eat these things. I am saying be aware that the tamasic foods are heavier and harder to digest, therefore they will make you feel low in energy. The rajasic foods are stimulating and will cause restlessness and a lack of focus. You will notice that sugar, wheat and alcohol are in both rajas and tamas. This is because they can initially energise and cause us to feel more rajasic, then they eventually lead to a more tamasic state after the rajasic effect has worn off, especially if consumed in excess.

A WORD ABOUT DIGESTION.

Agni is our digestive fire or an indicator of our digestive function. When our agni is functioning well we digest food easily and absorb all the nutrients needed to keep us healthy. When our agni is impaired we experience digestion problems, even a bit of heartburn is a sign that something is imbalanced in the agni. When it's out of balance we don't get all the nutrients we need on a cellular level so the bodymind becomes depleted. In addition the poorly digested food can hang around in the digestive system (which includes the stomach, small and large intestine) causing inflammation and toxins (ama) which lead to disease. A healthy happy agni means a healthy happy bodymind. Sattvic food, cleansing (see page 99) and cyclical living support good agni.

We begin eating with our senses, before we even put food anywhere near the mouth. The salivary glands in the mouth react to the stimulus of what we see and smell. This begins the digestion. This then lets the stomach know something will be coming along fairly soon and the bile gets secreted by the gall bladder into the stomach ready to digest. If we don't stop to look at or smell the food, if we shovel it into the body and swallow without fully chewing, this process doesn't work properly.

If we don't chew thoroughly we experience digestive problems. These issues can range from indigestion to gas and bloating. Over a prolonged period of time (several months and years), this leads to toxins (ama) building up in the system because the undigested food gets stuck and this causes stagnation and inflammation in the gut.

Couple that with food that isn't right for our body and you have even more for the digestion to cope with. This inflammation becomes the trigger for long term chronic dis-ease. I could go on, you get the idea. Look at your food, then smell it, and then please properly chew before you swallow. Don't take another mouthful until you have completely swallowed the mouthful you are eating, and so on.

It is important to eat sitting down. If we are standing up or walking the bodymind is confused. It knows we are moving so may perceive there is a threat. This is our natural survival response. When we are moving or standing we are usually in a heightened state of awareness. We need to be relaxed to digest properly.

REST AND DIGEST.

Sit down. Also please sit fully upright so your lovely, and quite frankly amazing, internal organs have space to do their job properly.

Our digestion is at its height in the middle of the day between 12 and 2pm. Therefore ideally eat your main meal of the day at this time and have a light supper by 7pm. If we are not digesting food properly we will not get then nutrients from the food we are eating. If we do not get nutrients from food we again create dis-ease.

FOOD IS OUR MEDICINE

In general terms in ayurveda we use very little onions and garlic, there are specific food guidelines for your constitutional state and the changing seasons. We always recommend eating locally sourced seasonal food as this is naturally the correct food for the climate you are living in, even if that is not your native land. For example, a banana will not grow in the UK, so I limit my intake of bananas (never in winter and only occasional in summer). When I am in South India, where bananas grow, I eat them all the time. Also limit raw food, especially in the evening as this is more difficult for the body to digest. Don't mix raw and cooked food as they digest at different rates. Fruit in general needs to be eaten alone, not with other foods. This because when mixed with other foods it can ferment as it's digested differently. Of course, in the West we are used to mixing fruit all the time so it can feel challenging to change this. If you're wanting to be very specific about your diet and to make adjustments according to you individual dosha balance then it's best to do this with a practitioner consultation as everyone is so individual.

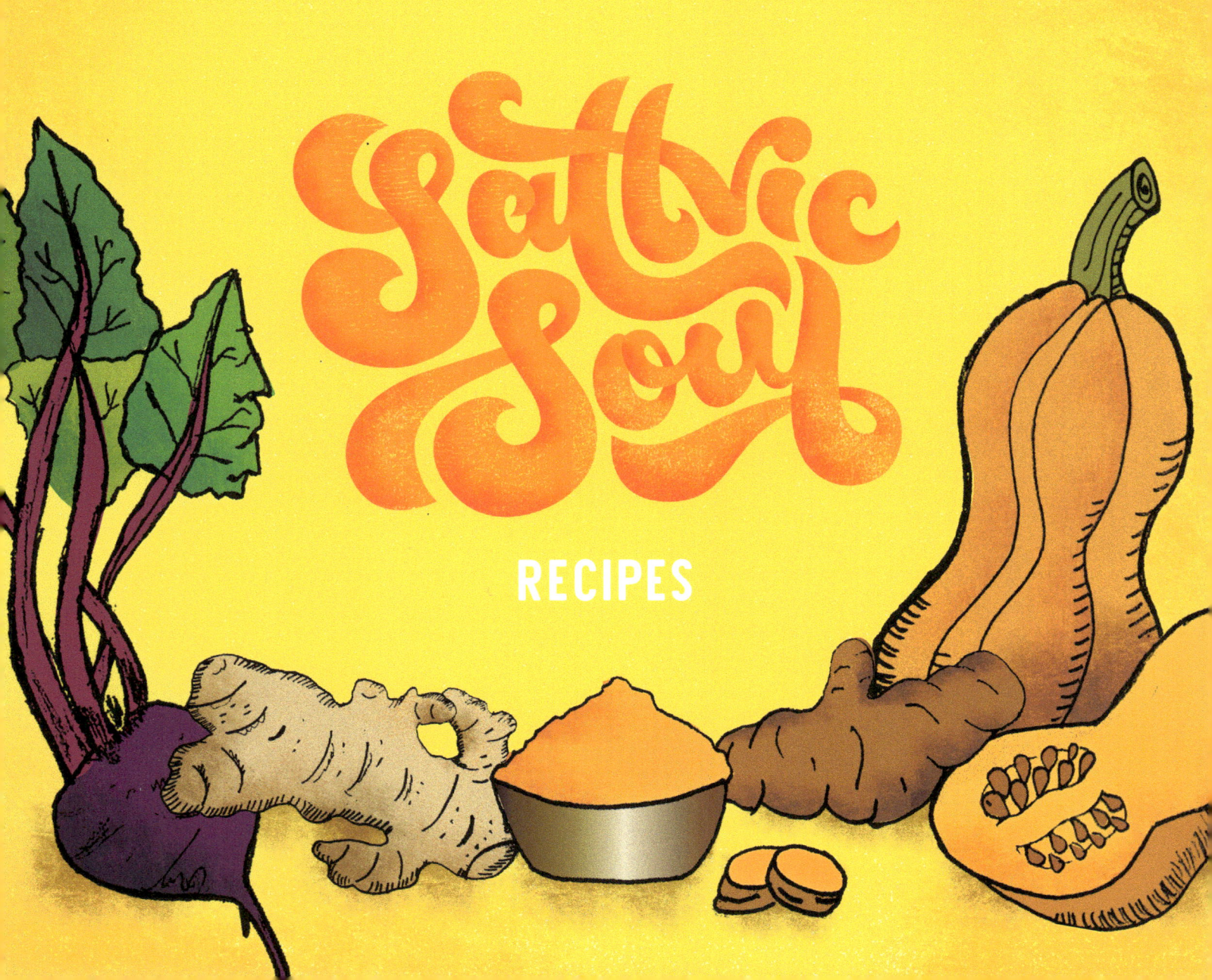

The little flame icon will let you know how long the recipe takes to prepare. Some things need a bit of preparation with 'soaking' the day before. Here is a general guide.

Ideally needs some soaking the day before so prepare a bit in advance, although final cooking may not take too long.

GET CREATIVE IN THE KITCHEN.

Lots of people wanted me to write a recipe book! This part is for those people, with love.

The recipes are all sattvic, they are in line with the principles of ayurveda mentioned above, with the occasional twist. I encourage you to use seasonal and locally sourced produce wherever possible. I have generally used coconut or sesame oils, but you can substitute with olive, hemp or sunflower oils or ghee (for more information on ghee see page 103). Personally I view recipes as an inspiration. I read them, then go off piste a bit and throw other stuff in and change things about, so please do use these recipes in this way.

All of these recipes serve around two people generously. They are all vegan, unless you use ghee or add dairy as occasionally suggested.

A note on heat in the body. If you have excess heat in the body, please avoid the more fiery and heating spices. Excess heat may show up as literally feeling hot in your body or being hot tempered, hot skin rashes, indigestion, gallbladder issues and liver inflammation. Each recipe highlights where this may be the case.

Prepare on the day, some time needed but relatively straightforward.

Really quick and simple.

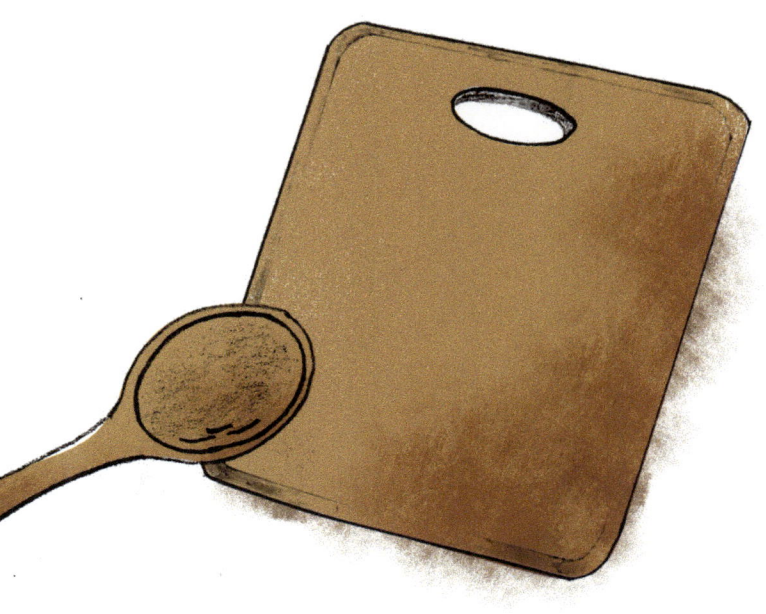

BREAKFAST.

Break......fast

This is the first meal of the day, obvious I know. It is therefore super important that it is simple, easy to digest and delicious. The below suggestions are all these things.

STEWED APPLE.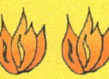

4 apples (cooking or eating apples)
1 inch ginger, grated
1 teaspoon cinnamon
4 medjool dates (remove stones and chop)
Rice syrup, maple syrup or local honey to taste (optional)

1. Peel and chop the apples and add to a non-stick pan with just a couple of cm of water.

2. Bring to simmer with the lid on and then add the ginger and cinnamon.

3. Gently stir, add the dates.

4. Keep simmering for 20 minutes, with a lid on. Stir occasionally throughout.

5. Check everything is nicely cooked and serve warm. It should be sweet enough with the dates, if not you can stir in some rice syrup, maple syrup or local honey.

PORRIDGE.

1 cup of porridge oats
2 cups of water, dairy or plant milk
1 teaspoon of local honey, or maple or rice syrup
1 tablespoon of mixed seeds, hemp, sesame, pumpkin, sunflower
2 teaspoons of ghee. hemp oil of fat of choice

Porridge churna or spice mix (you can make a larger quantity and keep ready mixed in a jar, this is enough for one sitting)
2 teaspoons turmeric
1 teaspoon cinnamon
½ teaspoon cardamon
½ teaspoon ginger

1. Cover the oats with water about 1cm over the top and soak overnight in a pan.

2. When you're ready for breakfast add either more water or a milk (dairy or plant based) to your soaked oats together with the spices.

3. Heat until gently bubbling.

4. Meanwhile dry toast the seeds in a pan until they smell toasty.

5. Stir in some fat, plus your sweetener.

6. Scatter seeds on top before serving.

BUCKWHEAT PANCAKES.

2 cups buckwheat flour
Water, to achieve desired consistency
1 teaspoon ground turmeric
1 teaspoon ground cinnamon
1 tablespoon coconut oil

1. Mix the flour and water with the turmeric and cinnamon. The consistency should be softly dropping, add the water slowly to achieve this.

2. Leave to stand for at least an hour or so, preferably overnight (at room temperature). It may have thickened whilst sitting so add a bit more water if required.

3. Heat the coconut oil in a non stick pan.

4. Drop the pancake mixture in so it makes little scotch pancake sized shapes.

5. Fry on one side then turn, making sure they are nicely browned on both sides.

6. Serve the pancakes piled up with maple or rice syrup.

MASALA OMELETTE.

A lovely spicy favourite for brunch! This recipes suggests courgette and cherry tomato but you can use any vegetables you choose, whatever is lying around or left over will do. Delicious with some ginger turmeric pickle and amazing Tibetan spicy raita (see page 77).

4 eggs
1 tablespoon coconut oil
1 courgette (chopped)
10 cherry tomatoes
1 good handful of spinach
1 red chilli (omit if you have heat tendencies in the body, see note on page 53)
1 handful of fresh chopped coriander
1 teaspoon ground turmeric
2 teaspoons garam masala
Pinch of salt

1. Heat the coconut oil a non-stick frying style pan on a fairly good heat.

2. Fry the courgettes until they begin to brown.

3. Whist the courgette is frying whisk the eggs together with the turmeric, garam masala and a pinch of salt.

4. Finely chop the spinach.

5. Cut the tomatoes into quarters.

6. When the courgette is brown add the tomatoes and stir fry for around a minute until they're nice and soft, but not mushy.

7. Stir in the spinach.

8. Mix the chopped coriander in with the egg mixture, stir well.

9. Pour the egg mixture into the pan and cook until the bottom is solid. Then place under a grill to cook the top.

10. Cut into generous wedges and serve.

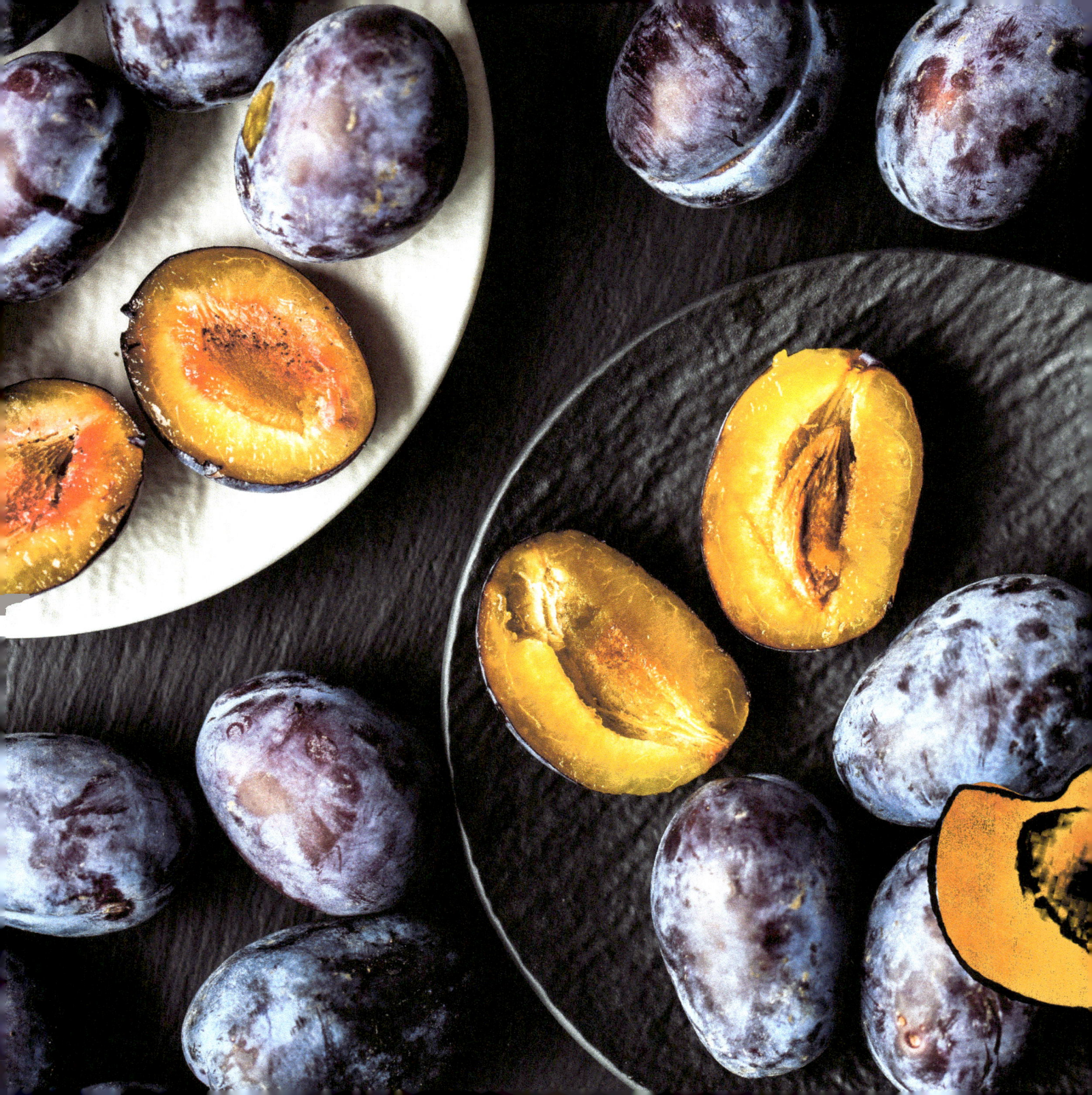

ROASTED STONEFRUIT.

8 stone fruit (any mix of peaches, nectarines, apricots, plums)
2 teaspoons balsamic vinegar (approx)
2 teaspoons maple syrup
1 teaspoon cinnamon

1. Heat the oven to 200°C.

2. Slice the stone fruit in half, remove the stones and place onto a baking tray cut side upwards.

3. Carefully drizzle a very small amount (about ¼ teaspoon per fruit maximum) of the balsamic vinegar and then the maple syrup over the fruit, just a drop or two on each piece of fruit is plenty.

4. Sprinkle over the cinnamon.

5. Bake in the oven for 30 minutes. The fruit should caramelise and the balsamic vinegar and maple syrup will create a deep burgundy sticky sauce.

6. Place the fruit onto serving plates and pour the sauce over.

POACHED PEARS.

4 pears
4 cardamom pods (cracked open)
4 cloves
1 cinnamon stick
2 teaspoons rosewater
1 inch ginger, grated
1 tablespoon maple syrup
500ml water

1. Cut the pears into quarters and remove the hard centre. No need to peel.

2. Add the spice, rosewater, maple syrup and enough water for the pears to poach into a wide pan.

3. Bring this mixture the gently to simmer then add the pears.

4. Simmer until cooked, 15-20 minutes depending on the ripeness of the pears.

5. Serve warm with the fragrant liquid poured over.

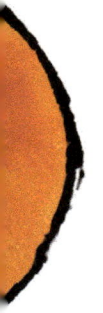
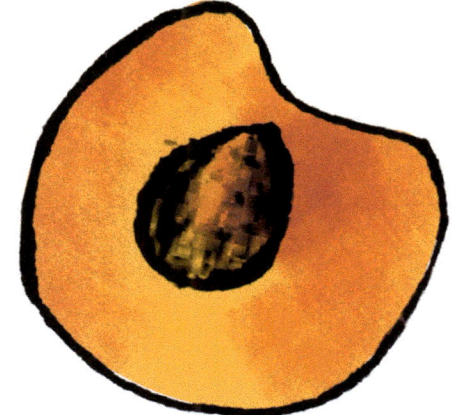

MAIN COURSES.

GREEN TEA SALAD.

I discovered this in a small Burmese restaurant the night before I flew back to the UK from New Zealand in 2010. The mixture of flavours blew me away! So I made it my business to find the recipe. This is definitely a very ritualistic process! It is so incredibly delicious, your efforts and patience are well rewarded!

1 good sized bag of greens of choice, kale or rocket are good
200ml tamari soya sauce
4 limes, juiced
2 inches fresh ginger, grated
4 tablespoons green tea
Pinch or two of himalayan salt
1 cup desiccated coconut
1 cup sesame seeds
1 cup cashew nuts

1. Preheat the oven to 150°C

2. Finely shred the greens of choice really, really finely so they're about the size of grated carrot, easy to pick up with a fork. If you are using tougher greens like kale then sprinkle the salt onto them and massage gently until they 'relax' a little. There is no need to do this with softer salad type greens.

3. Add the grated ginger to the tamari sauce, green tea and the juice of the limes. Soak for at least two hours, ideally make it in the morning and leave it all day.

4. Mix the sesame seeds and desiccated coconut together and spread thinly on a baking sheet.

5. Bake in an oven at 150°C for five minutes or until toasted, keep an eye on them so they don't burn.

6. Spread the cashew nuts onto a baking sheet and pop into the same oven for ten minutes or until toasted, again keep an eye on them.

7. Leave the coconut, seeds and nuts to go cold.

8. After at least a couple of hours of everything cooling, relaxing and marinading, begin again.

9. Rinse the greens so the salt is removed (if necessary) and pat dry.

10. Spread the shredded greens thinly over a large serving plate.

11. Scatter the coconut, seeds and cashews.

12. Strain / sieve the dressing mixture and take the ginger pulp and green tea leaves and squeeze every last bit out of it all. Pour the dressing all over the leaf seed coconut mixture.

13. Allow to sit for fifteen minutes or so then serve. It's amazing!

Delicious healthy meal involving Green Tea salad
Using the salad as a base on the plate, layer with some Tibetan spicy sauce, ume radishes (see page 71) around the edge, take some fried tempeh or tofu and pile it in the middle, garnish with sprouting seeds (radish seeds if possible) on the top.

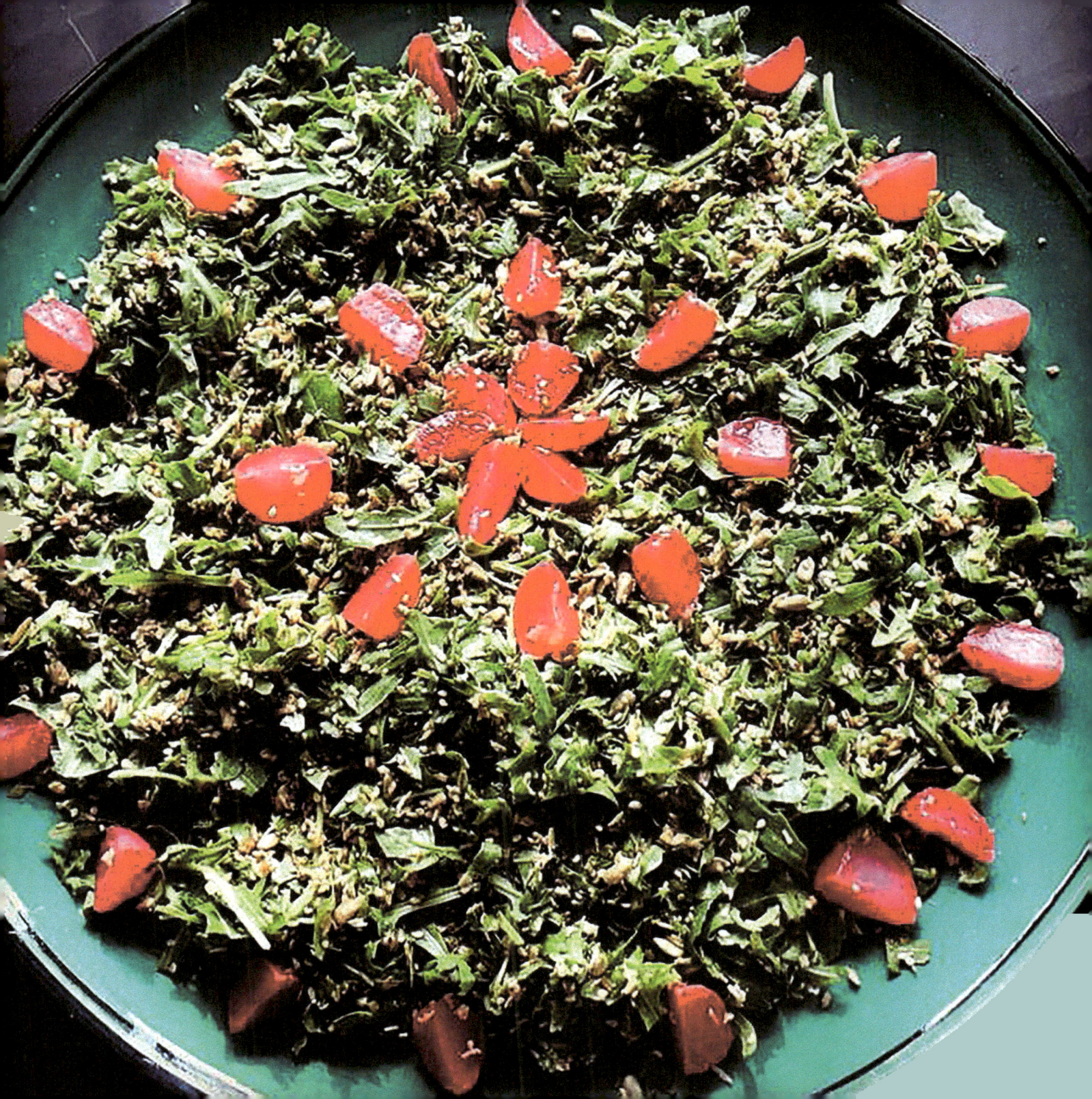

BOMBAY MIX SALAD.

This is delicious, it's a bit of a take on street food from India. Be sure to add the bombay mix at the last minute before serving so it doesn't go soggy.

3 cups bombay mix
1 handful peanuts, roasted then cooled
2 large potatoes, peeled, boiled and chopped into tiny cubes
2 shallots, finely chopped
2 large tomatoes, finely chopped
1 handful of coriander, finely chopped
2 green chilies, finely chopped (optional, omit if you have heat tendencies in the body)
1 tablespoon tamarind chutney

1. In a large bowl mix the peanuts, potato, shallot, tomato, coriander, and green chilies together with the chutney.

2. When ready to serve add and stir through the bombay mix and eat immediately.

KALE AND BROCCOLI WITH SIMPLE SATAY STYLE DRESSING.

This is delectable on its own or as a side dish. You could also make the tofu and kale (next recipe) and incorporate the broccoli with it and exchange the tahini dressing (see page 75) for this one. I also use the stalks of the broccoli, which taste incredibly sweet and delicious.

1 bag of kale (any type is okay), big stalks removed and leaves torn into bite sized pieces
2 large heads and stalks of broccoli, chopped into small bite-sized pieces
1 teaspoon sea salt (don't be tempted to use more)
½ cup tamari soy sauce
1 cup peanut butter
1 red chilli (omit if you have heat tendencies in the body)

1. Lightly steam the broccoli, for four to five minutes keeping it vibrantly green and alive, leave to cool

2. Sprinkle the kale with the salt and massage it gently until it 'relaxes' a little. Rinse the salt off and pat dry.

3. Mix the broccoli and kale together.

4. Blend together the soy sauce, peanut butter and chilli with water to make a sauce the consistency of a thick pouring cream.

5. Pile up the broccoli and kale and pour the dressing over.

6. This is really good served with toasted tamari seeds (see page 74) sprinkled over.

TOFU AND KALE WITH TAHINI DRESSING.

2 packs of smoked firm tofu, cut into smallish cubes
1 bag of Kale (preferably the curly type),
large stalks removed and torn into bite sized pieces
2 good sized cooked beetroot,
chopped into smallish equal sized pieces
1 cup pomegranate seeds
1 cup sprouted seeds of choice
1 cup toasted pumpkin seeds (see page 74)
1 inch fresh ginger, grated
1 red chilli, finely chopped
1 tablespoon tamari soy sauce
2 tablespoons tahini (light)
1 lemon, juiced

1. Chop everything and have it to hand to make your life easier.

2. Take a wok and heat with a little oil, hemp or rapeseed oil is nice to use here.

3. Add the grated ginger root, chopped chilli, cubed tofu and the tamari soy sauce.

4. Cook for around 3-4 minutes until the tofu is a little browned, add the kale. The kale will quickly wilt, you want to retain its vibrant green colour and not overcook it so this will only take a minute.

5. Quickly add the beetroot, half of the pomegranate and pumpkin and sprouted seeds and stir all together.

6. Mix the tahini and lemon juice together, add water and keep mixing until you achieve a double cream type consistency. (Make the dressing at the last minute as if you leave it sitting it will thicken).

7. Pile the mixture of seeds, kale, tofu and beetroot onto plates. Pour the tahini dressing over the top. Then pile on top the remaining pomegranate seeds, toasted pumpkin seeds and sprouting seeds.

8. Eat immediately and feel very virtuous and healthy!

LEMON COURGETTES.

2 courgettes
1 lemon
3 garlic cloves (use less or omit if you have heat tendencies in the body)
2 tablespoons olive oil
Pinch of salt

1. Preheat the oven to 200°C

2. Slice the courgettes in half lengthways then into thin half moon shapes.

3. Take each garlic clove and smash it roughly with the side of a knife.

4. Put the courgette and garlic into a baking tray and drizzle with olive oil and a pinch of salt. Move the courgette around and coat it in the oil.

5. Cut the lemon into eight pieces and distribute around the baking tray.

6. Roast for around 40 minutes or until soft and slightly brown at the edges.

POTATOES.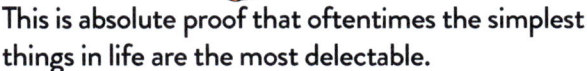

This is absolute proof that oftentimes the simplest things in life are the most delectable.

3 medium sized potatoes per person
2 tablespoons of olive oil
Generous pinch of salt

1. Preheat the oven to 200°C

2. Wash the potatoes and pat them dry. Prick them with a fork and place in a baking tray

3. Drizzle the potatoes with olive oil, just enough that you can rub it into the skin but not so much that they're swimming in it.

4. Sprinkle with a good quality sea salt and rub this into the skin.

5. Place into the oven for around one hour, skins will be slightly crisp, insides soft.

6. Split open and drizzle more olive oil over the insides.

7. Serve with other dishes, like the baked beans (see page 63). They're also truly delicious on their own and with a very good dressing like the hemp seed mayo (see page 75).

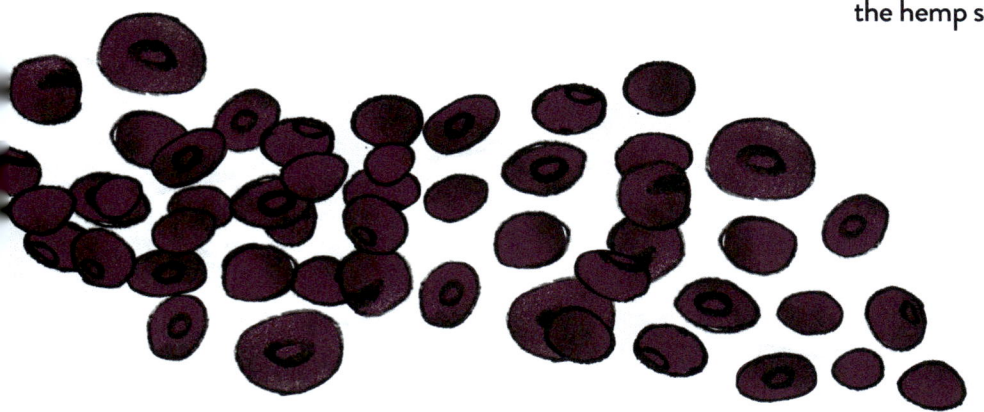

BEAN CHILLI.

This recipe requires some pre-planning but it is worth it. The pre-cooking plus the walking away gives a delicious depth of flavour that only comes with patience and relaxation time taken well.
You can substitute the dried beans and use tinned instead. I really like this with short grain brown rice but you can serve it with whatever you like, of course. And it is even more tasty and satisfying the following day.

3 sticks celery
3 teaspoons smoked paprika
2 teaspoons cumin seed
2 red chillis (more if you like it spicy)
1 cup dried aduki beans, soaked and pre-cooked (or 1 tin)
1 cup dried kidney beans, soaked and pre-cooked (or 1 tin)
1 cup dried black beans, soaked and pre-cooked (or 1 tin)
1 tin of chopped tomatoes
4 tablespoons tomato puree
1 teaspoon asafoetida (hing)
Pinch of salt (to taste)
100g dark chocolate
1 tablespoon coconut oil

1. Sauté the celery in the coconut oil until it's soft.

2. Add in the chopped chilli, paprika, cumin seeds and asafoetida, stir for a couple of minutes.

3. Add chopped tomatoes and tomato puree, bring to simmer.

4. Stir in the beans, if you need more liquid add some water.

5. Simmer for 10 minutes then turn the whole thing off and walk away for at least two hours. Do something wonderfully relaxing with this time, have a hot bath, do a yoga nidra, go for a walk in nature, read a good book, meditate, do some quality daydreaming. Use this time very wisely.

6. Return and bring to a gentle simmer again. Once simmering, add the dark chocolate and stir in until it's all dissolved. Add salt to taste and serve.

BAKED BEANS.

Delicious proper baked beans! Lovely eaten on a cold autumn day, excellent the next day (allowing spices to intermingle) with a baked potato.

400g cooked haricot beans or similar
1 tin chopped tomatoes
2 tablespoons tomato puree
2 tablespoons molasses
2 teaspoons smoked paprika
2 red chillies chopped (optional, omit if you have heat tendencies in the body)
2 teaspoons ground cumin
Salt to taste

1. Preheat the oven to 200°C

2. Mix everything together and pour it into an ovenproof baking tray.

3. Cover with a lid or some foil and bake at 200°C for 30 minutes.

4. Remove from the oven, stir and serve.

ADUKI BEETROOT STEW.

This is really so delicious and very easy. It has the advantage of making you feel very virtuous.
It's also incredibly good for the liver. Delicious with some kind of mash like celeriac and mustard or with short grain brown rice and greens. Grounding and sweetly nourishing. You need to pre-prepare the beans by soaking and pressure cooking or substitute and use tinned.

4 sticks celery, finely chopped
2 carrots, finely chopped
400g dried aduki beans,
soaked and pre-cooked (or 2 tins)
2 fresh beetroots, peeled and grated
2 teaspoons fennel seed
2 teaspoons cumin seed
1 teaspoon asafoetida (hing)
3 cups vegetable stock
Salt to taste
1 tablespoon coconut oil

1. Sauté the carrot and celery in the coconut oil until soft.

2. Add the cumin and fennel seeds and sauté for a couple more minutes until they smell aromatic.

3. Add the aduki beans (already cooked) and stir in, then add a little veg stock until the beans are almost, but not quite, covered.

4. Simmer for ten minutes.

5. Add the grated beetroot and simmer for a further ten minutes so the beetroot gently softens and is cooked.

6. Add salt to taste and serve.

AROMATIC SWEET POTATO AND TOFU.

2 medium sweet potatoes, peeled and chopped into square pieces
1 block smoked firm tofu, chopped into square pieces
1 tablespoon sesame oil
2 large red Chillies, (optional, omit if you have heat tendencies in the body)
2 teaspoon ground turmeric, or 2 inches of fresh, grated
1 teaspoon asafoetida (hing)
2 inches fresh ginger, grated
1 tin coconut milk (full fat)
200 ml water
1 lime, juiced
1 bunch fresh coriander, roughly chopped
Black pepper
Salt to taste

1. A couple of hours (or more) beforehand cut the tofu into cubes and marinate in half of the turmeric and grated ginger with the sesame oil.

2. When you're ready to start cooking place all ingredients apart from the sweet potatoes, tofu and fresh coriander into a large saucepan, bring to the boil stirring then reduce the heat and simmer for five minutes.

3. Add the sweet potato, mix well and simmer for 20 minutes or until the potatoes are tender.

4. Add the diced marinated tofu for the last ten minutes.

5. Garnish at the last minute with the fresh coriander and serve.

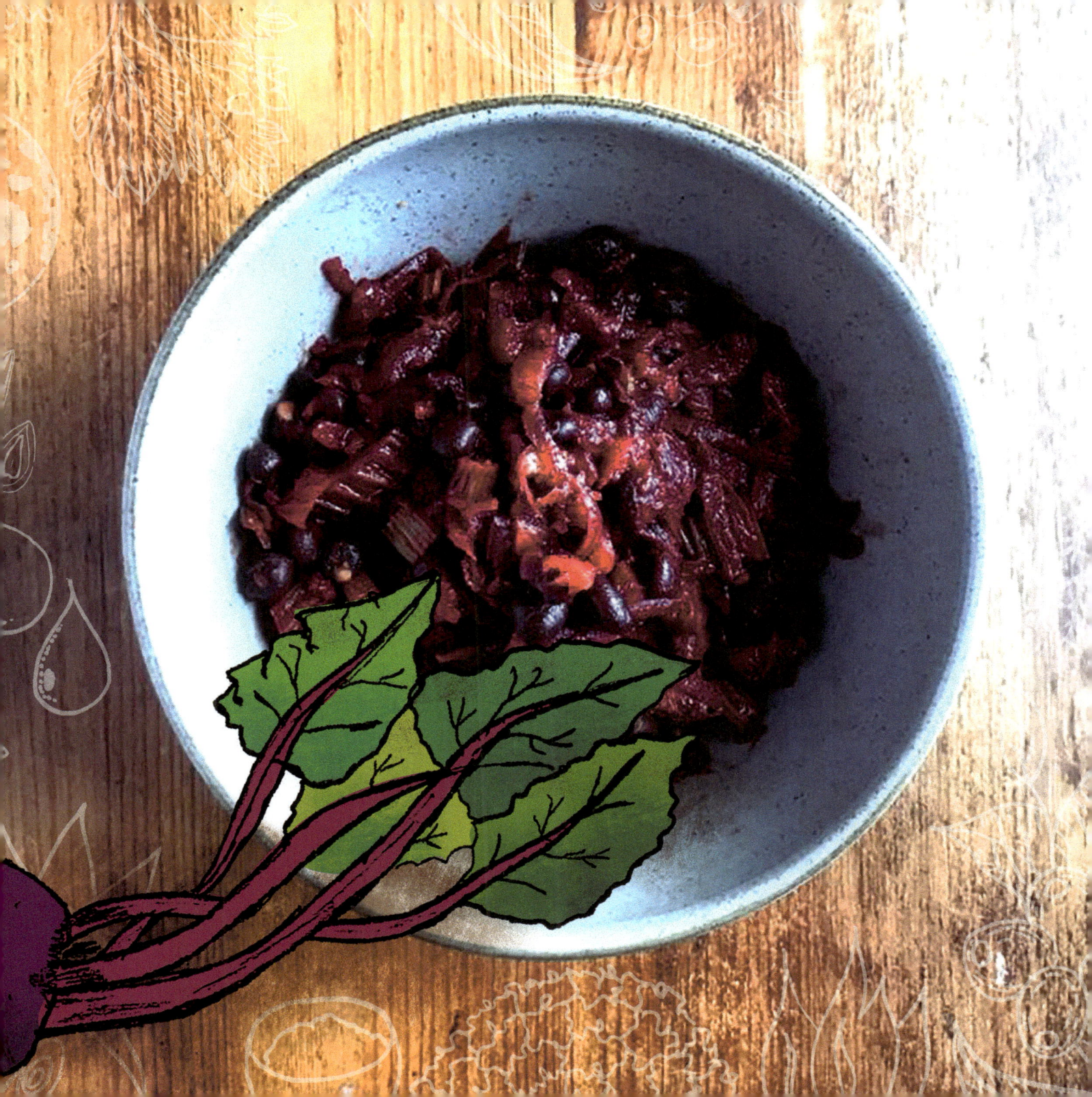

VEGAN AYURVEDIC CASSOULET.

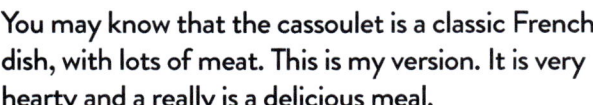

You may know that the cassoulet is a classic French dish, with lots of meat. This is my version. It is very hearty and a really is a delicious meal.

1 leek, finely chopped
1 fennel bulb, finely chopped
2 aubergines, chopped into small squares and roasted at 200°C for 45 minutes
½ cup dried red lentils
2 cups dried then cooked or 1 tin of black eyed beans (or other beans of choice)
2 cloves garlic, finely chopped (optional)
1 big jar of tomato passata
Either 2 tablespoons dried or 1 cupful of mixed fresh, parsley and oregano
3 cups breadcrumbs, (stale but good bread broken down into crumbs is best)
1 ½ cups engivita yeast flakes
2 cups sunflower seeds
1 cup olive oil
Salt to taste

1. Ensure you have all ingredients to hand and pre-prepared, pre-cooked, chopped up where needed, with either a hob to oven pot, or a pan plus an oven dish.

2. Pre heat the oven to 180°C.

3. Pour half the olive oil into the pan and sauté the chopped fennel and leek. Once they are soft add the garlic (if using).

4. Add the red lentils, passata and 1 cup of water so the lentils can cook. Leave them to simmer for around 20 minutes, stirring occasionally. Add more water during cooking if needed.

5. Once the lentils are cooked, they will go mushy and lose their shape, they will also expand so do keep a watchful eye.

6. Stir in the other beans and pre-cooked aubergine.

7. Mix everything together until it is well combined. Stir in just a quarter of the herbs and salt to taste. Decant the whole lot into an oven dish.

8. In a bowl mix together the breadcrumbs, yeast flakes, sunflower seeds, remaining herbs and roughly a tablespoon of olive oil (just enough oil to lightly coat everything but not make it swimming).

9. Take one third of the breadcrumb mixture and cover the top of the beans in the baking dish. Place it into the oven until it is crispy on top, around 20 minutes.

10. Take it out of the oven and stir in the topping. Repeat this process, cover it with another third of the breadcrumb mixture, bake until crispy and take out and stir in the topping again.

11. The third time don't stir the topping in, it's ready to eat!

12. Great served with greens or a salad.

SUPER SIMPLE FAST FOOD.

The next few recipes are super simple! They use some basic store cupboard ingredients and whatever leftovers you might have to hand. Ideal if you're busy and don't have much time.

COCONUT CURRY SAUCE.

This is a basic simple sauce, to which you can add anything you choose.

1 tin of coconut milk (full fat)
2 teaspoons ground turmeric
2-4 teaspoons garam masala (depending on taste)
1 teaspoon asafoetida (hing)
Fresh coriander, a good handful
Salt (to taste)
1 tablespoon coconut oil

1. Make a paste from the turmeric, garam masala, asafoetida, fresh coriander and salt.

2. Sauté the paste in coconut oil for just a couple of minutes.

3. Add the coconut milk.

4. Simmer everything together gently and add whatever vegetables you like.

5. Continue to simmer until the vegetables are cooked and then serve.

VEGETABLE RICE.

This is a dish that is generally put together with leftovers, so quantities are estimated and will vary depending on what you have available.

2 cups of mixed fresh vegetables
1 cup cooked rice
1 teaspoon ground turmeric
1 teaspoon garam masala
Handful of fresh coriander (if available)

1. Take a selection of whatever vegetables you like and chop them finely.

2. Separate any green leafy vegetables from any root vegetables.

3. Sauté the root vegetables in coconut oil until you are satisfied they are cooked.

4. Add the rice.

5. Stir in turmeric, garam masala, add the fresh coriander if you have some.

6. If using greens (spinach for example) add this after the rice and stir in at the very end so it retains its fresh green demeanour.

STIR FRIED GREENS.

This is simple and delicious as a side dish or with kitchari.

1 courgette
2 sticks celery, finely chopped
1 fennel bulb
1 leek
1 head and stalk of broccoli
1 handful of French type green beans, chopped into short pieces
1 handful of kale, variety of your choice, roughly torn into small pieces
1 teaspoon fennel seeds
1 teaspoon cumin seeds
1 teaspoon coriander seeds
1 teaspoon ground turmeric
1 inch fresh ginger, grated
1 tablespoon ghee or coconut oil

1. Chop the courgette, leek, fennel, celery and stalk of the broccoli into small bite size pieces.

2. Sauté in either ghee or coconut oil with the spices (excluding the ginger) for 15 - 20 minutes until soft.

3. Add the ginger, finely chopped green beans and broccoli florets, continue to sauté for a further five minutes.

4. Add the kale. Stir in to wilt but remain green and serve.

POTATOES AND GREENS.

Enough potatoes for two people, cut into small sized cubes
1 good size bag of spinach, chard or similar, torn into bite sized pieces
250g bag of frozen peas
2 teaspoons garam masala
2 teaspoons turmeric
1 teaspoon asafoetida (hing)
1 tablespoon coconut oil
1 pack of paneer or feta cheese (optional)

1. In a large saucepan sauté the spices in the oil for 2 minutes until they smell aromatic.

2. Add water to about halfway up the saucepan, bring to simmer then add the potatoes until they are almost cooked, about 20 minutes.

3. Add the peas and continue to simmer for further 5 minutes.

4. At the last minute stir in the spinach.

5. If you eat dairy you can have this with paneer or feta cheese, stir through at the last minute before serving.

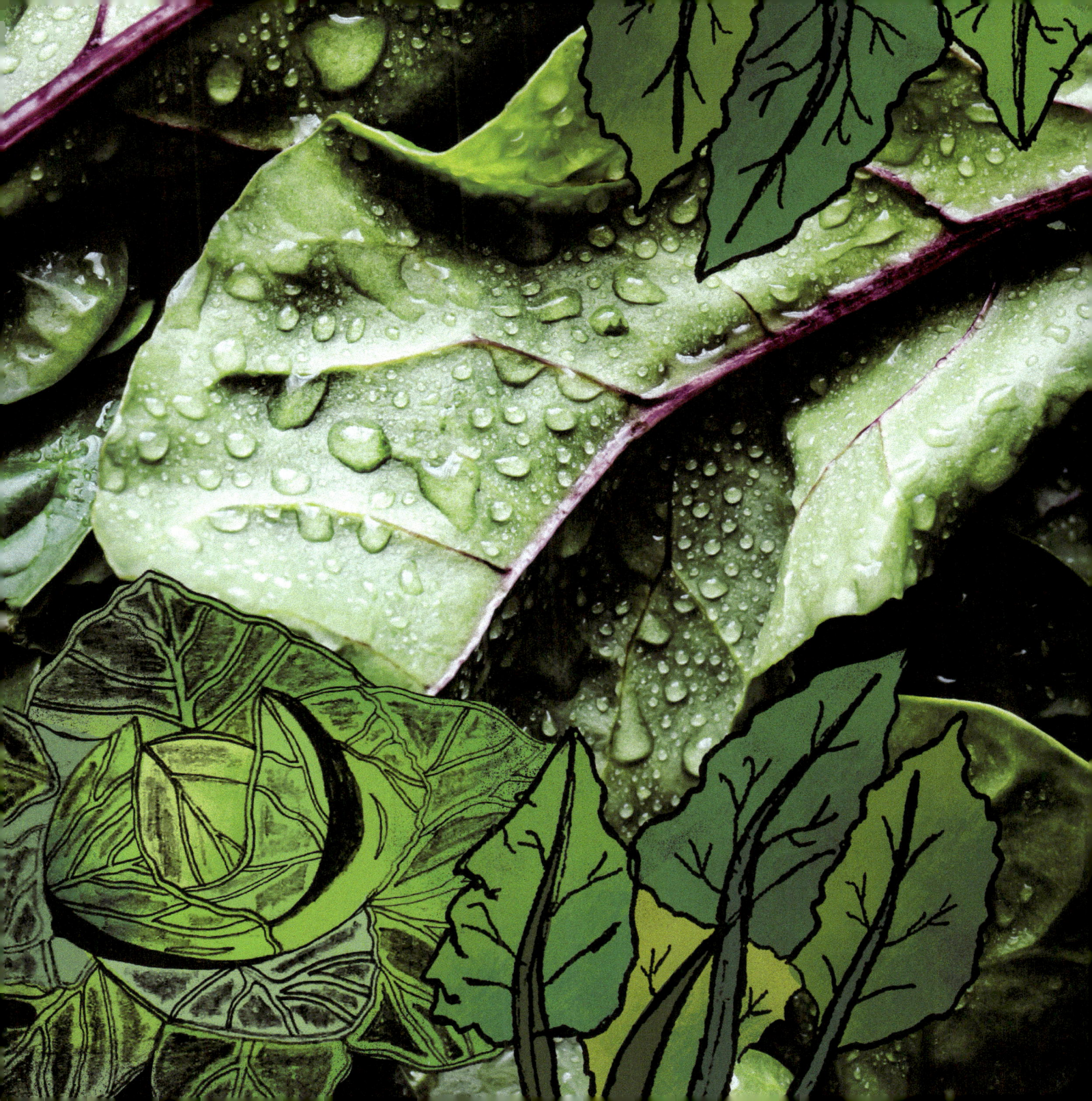

ROAST ROOT VEG.

This is lovely and grounding for autumn.

Selection of 3 or 4 root vegetables per person, for example, squash, beetroot, parsnips, sweet potato, carrots
2 teaspoons ground cinnamon
1 teaspoon ground paprika
1 pack halloumi cheese (optional)
1 pack plain tofu (optional)
1 cup toasted pumpkin seeds (see page 74)
1 pomegranate fruit, seeds
Handful each of fresh coriander, parsley and mint (roughly chopped)
2 tablespoons sunflower oil

1. Take the root vegetables and chop them to even size pieces. Top tip: Par boil the beetroots first for 30 minutes as they can take ages to cook.

2. Pour over the sunflower oil and rub in the cinnamon and paprika.

3. Roast for around 45 minutes, until cooked.

4. Add halloumi or tofu for the final 15 minutes if you like.

5. Serve with pomegranate seeds and toasted pumpkin seeds, freshly chopped mint, parsley and coriander. Lovely with a tahini dressing (see page 75).

BEETROOT SAUTE.

4 beetroots, grated
1 inch fresh ginger, grated
2 teaspoons black onion seed (nigella)
1 cup desiccated coconut
1 cup sesame seeds
1 tablespoon sesame oil

1. Put the sesame oil into a pan and add the nigella seed, fry for a couple of minutes.

2. Add the beetroot and ginger. Keep stirring occasionally to softly cook the beetroot. The beetroot will be cooked after five minutes.

3. Add the coconut and sesame seeds for the final five minutes and stir in.

INDIAN ROAST CHICKPEAS.

Chickpeas and cumin are the best of friends, especially with a little salt.

2 tins chickpeas or 2 cups dried soaked, cooked chickpeas
2 teaspoons cumin powder
½ teaspoon salt
1 teaspoon turmeric
Sunflower oil

1. Pre heat oven to 180°C.

2. Lay the chickpeas on a on baking sheet and drizzle over a little sunflower oil, just enough to coat.

3. Add the spices, rubbing the oil and spices well in. If possible leave this to marinate overnight.

4. Roast for 15 minutes. Serve as a snack or with a main meal.

YUMMY CONDIMENTS AND LITTLE SNACKS.

These things add to your meal, people are usually impressed and wonder how you've made them, they are all super simple.

GOMASSIO (SESAME SALT).

Makes a small jarful which will keep for several weeks. This is great if you like a lot of salt on food but want to avoid eating too much salt. My absolute favourite combination is to use black sesame seeds and Himalayan pink salt, it just feels a bit sexy and special, but do play around and use whatever combination you prefer.

20 teaspoons of sesame seeds (you can use regular or black sesame seeds, sometimes called nigella)
½ a teaspoon of salt (preferably a good rock salt or Himalayan pink salt)

1. Gently warm, but do not overheat, a large frying pan or wok.

2. Toast the sesame seeds, keep gently moving them around with a wooden spoon. until they smell toasty. It will take around 15 minutes. You should be able to pick one up and crumble it between your thumb and forefinger, if you can't crumble the seed keep going and be patient.

3. Once toasted to crumbling point tip the sesame seeds into a good solid pestle and mortar.

4. Take ½ teaspoon of salt and gently heat it in the same pan for two minutes, just to take any dampness out.

5. Add the salt to the seeds in the pestle and mortar.

6. Grind the seeds and the salt together. It gives off a gorgeous aroma as you do this so inhale deeply! Grind it all so that the seeds are a rough dust consistency. You can grind until its really fine if you like but personally I like to keep a few seeds whole as well.

7. Store in an airtight jar and use as you wish as a salty condiment to all food.

UME RADISHES.

1 small bag or bunch of radishes of choice
½ small bottle of ume plum seasoning

1. Slice the radishes into quarters and place into a small pan with the ume.

2. Add water to just about cover.

3. Bring to simmer for 10 minutes then switch off the heat and leave to sit in the cooking liquid for about 30 minutes.

4. Drain off the liquid and serve as a meal accompaniment / pickle, or store in the liquid in a jar for up to one week.

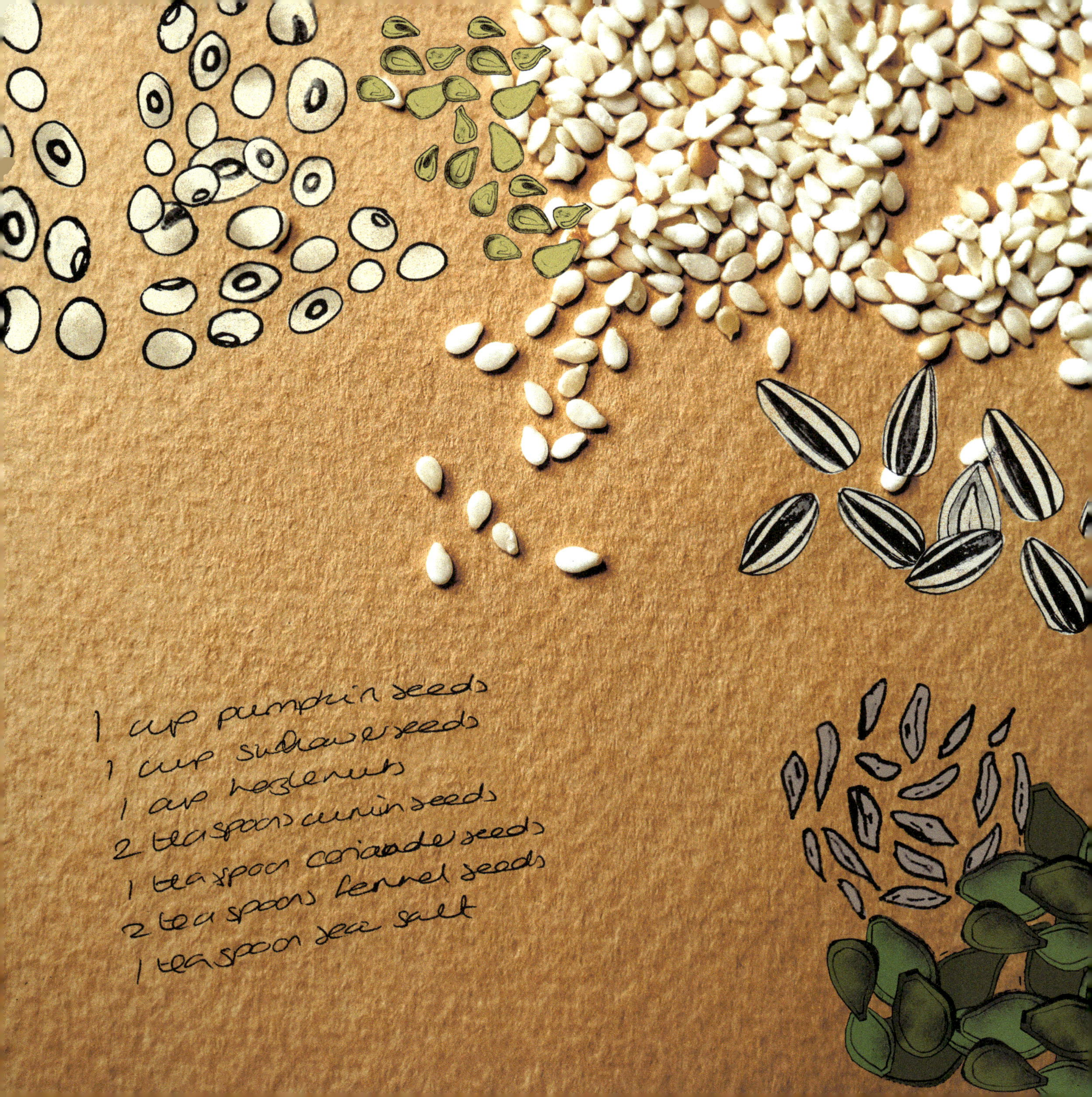

1 cup pumpkin seeds
1 cup sunflower seeds
1 cup hazelnuts
2 teaspoons cumin seeds
1 teaspoon coriander seeds
2 teaspoons fennel seeds
1 teaspoon sea salt

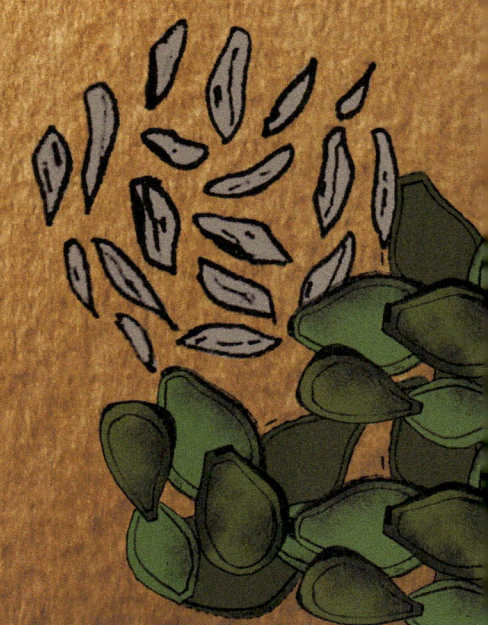

DUKKAH (DELICIOUS NUTTY HEALTHY SNACK).

Absolutely delicious with fresh bread. Have the bread nicely chopped into chunks and then a bowl with olive oil and balsamic and another bowl full of the dukkah. Dip the bread into the olive oil and balsamic mix then into the dukkah. Very moreish!

1 cup pumpkin seeds
1 cup sunflower seeds
1 cup hazelnuts
2 teaspoons cumin seeds
1 teaspoon coriander seeds
2 teaspoons fennel seeds
1 teaspoon sea salt

1. Heat the oven to 200°C.

2. Dry roast the hazelnuts in the oven for 10 minutes, until brown but not burned. Leave to cool.

3. Toast the seeds (separately from one another, see toasted seeds recipe on page 74) in a dry frying pan until they smell divinely toasty and are brownish. Leave to cool.

4. Toast the spices in the same way and leave to cool.

5. Place all the cooled ingredients together in a food processor and blend until it is the consistency of coarse breadcrumbs and well mixed together.

6. Store in an airtight jar for up to four weeks.

GINGER TURMERIC PICKLE.

This is so simple and yet so delicious and so good for you! Pickle with food is said to aid the digestion, plus the benefits of ginger and turmeric are so incredible they should be an essential part of any diet.

4 inches fresh ginger root
3 inches fresh turmeric root
2 lemons, juiced
1 teaspoon himalayan salt

1. Peel the ginger and turmeric. You can do this however you like, but if you use a knife you will lose a lot of the root. **Top tip:** Use a teaspoon to scrape the thin skin from the roots, and you will find you lose none of the valuable medicinal root.

2. Thinly chop the roots into matchstick shapes, as thin as you possibly can. Use it as a patience practice, be meditative, it will be worth it.

3. Place into a clean jar.

4. Pour over the juice of the lemons and add the salt making sure the chopped roots are just about covered.

5. Mix it all up.

6. Eaten immediately it is really delicious, or it can be kept in the fridge for a few weeks, whereupon the potency simply increases day by day.

TAMARI SEEDS.

These make a delicious and healthy snack, they can be used in salads or sprinkled with abandon as you wish on most savoury foods. Sunflower and pumpkin seeds are my seeds of choice.

Sunflower seeds help improve cholesterol levels, promote healthy detoxification, support skin health, are a good source of protein, assist with cancer prevention, manage high blood pressure and help to control blood sugar.

Pumpkin seeds are full of protein and healthy fats, they contain antioxidants that help fight disease and reduce inflammation, they can help with symptoms of enlarged prostate, are high in magnesium (which helps to control blood pressure, reduce risk of heart disease, maintain healthy bones and regulate blood sugar as well as helping improve sleep), they reduce blood pressure and increase good cholesterol.

If you're wanting to do both types of seeds please toast them separately. Firstly they 'perform' at slightly differing time scales and its also just somehow more satisfying to do them separately and to store them separately. If you consider the seeds from an energetic perspective, they're quite different. The sunflower grows up and out towards the light and is at its height in midsummer in the heat. The pumpkin grows low on the ground and is harvested in the autumn. Therefore the sunflower has an above ground, light and airy, fiery kind of quality and the pumpkin has more of a grounded, low lying, relaxed and heavy quality. This is also worth considering when using them in food and what effect you may wish to look for from the food you are ingesting and digesting.

200g pumpkin or sunflower seeds
2 teaspoons tamari soy sauce

1. Warm (do not overheat) a large frying pan or wok.

2. Place the chosen seeds in the pan. Do not then wander off. As soon as you become distracted or diverted they can burn. This is an exercise of patience. Keep gently turning the seeds in the pan. They will give off a lovely toasty aroma and go browner once they are done. Keep your nerve and get them as brown as you can.

3. Put the soy sauce into a bowl and, whilst still hot, tip the seeds into the bowl to make a satisfying hissing sound. Toss them around in the sauce until they all have a thin coating. Leave them to cool then stir again as they will stick together a little.

4. Store in an airtight jar and use within 2 weeks.

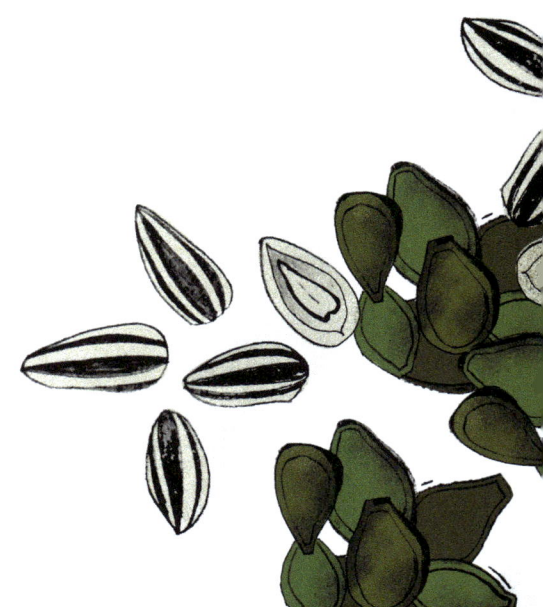

DRESSINGS AND DIPS.

Most of these dressing can be made either in a blender or by putting into a jar and giving a good shake or by mixing with a wooden spoon in a bowl. They can all be stored for a few days.

CLASSIC

2 lemons, juiced
Olive oil

1. Juice the lemons.
2. Mix with the same amount of olive oil.
3. Serve - simple and delicious!

TAHINI AND LEMON

1 tablespoon tahini
1 lemon, juiced

1. Mix together and add water to desired consistency, that of pouring cream.

OILY MUSTARD DRESSING

2 tablespoons olive oil
2 tablespoons balsamic vinegar or 1 lemon, juiced
1 teaspoon mustard, either wholegrain or French dijon

1. Mix together and serve.

HEMP SEED MAYO
(blender only)

1 cup hemp seeds
1 lemon, juiced
1 garlic clove roughly chopped (omit if you have heat tendencies in the body)
1 teaspoon mustard, French dijon is best
Water to give desired consistency
1 tablespoon yeast flakes (optional, add if you require a cheesy flavour)

1. Put everything apart from the water into a blender and whizz together.
2. Add the water slowly until you get the desired consistency. It can be a thick mayo, a thinner creamy dressing or anywhere in between.

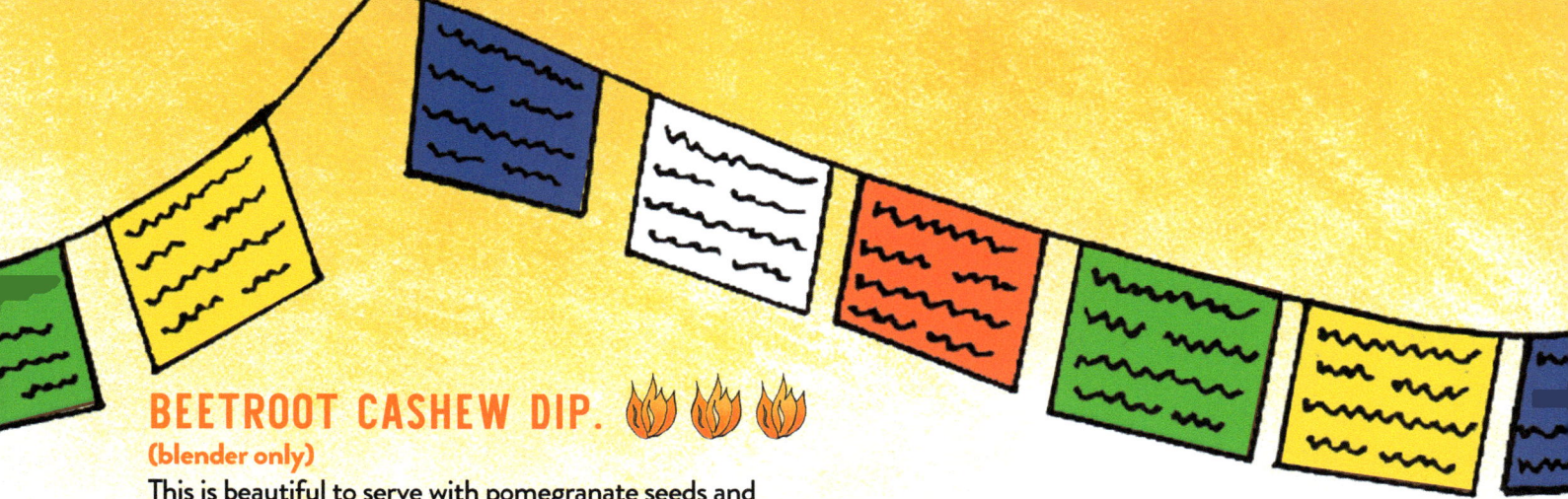

BEETROOT CASHEW DIP.
(blender only)

This is beautiful to serve with pomegranate seeds and caraway seeds on top in a lovely dish. It is delicious as a cheese or spread alternative, with salad, as a snack, part of tapas, use as you wish!

4 good size fresh beetroots
2 cups cashews
1 tablespoon caraway seeds (gently toast these in a dry frying pan to bring out the oil and more flavour)
1 tablespoon pomegranate molasses (optional)

1. The day before, prepare by soaking the cashews and leaving in cold water overnight. If you forget to do this then pour boiling water on them and leave for a minimum of one hour.

2. Pressure cook the beetroot for 15 minutes or boil in a pan for an hour, leave to cool (this can be done the day before), or buy ready cooked.

3. When you are ready to make the dip take the cooked beetroot and press the skins so they slip off, it is very satisfying!

4. Roughly chop the beets and put them into a food processor.

5. Drain and rinse the cashew nuts and add these to the food processor.

6. Add the pomegranate molasses, if using, and caraway seeds, blend until smooth.

TURMERIC DRESSING

2 lemons, juiced
1 inch fresh ginger, grated
2 inches fresh turmeric root, grated
3 tablespoons sesame oil
1 tablespoon apple cider vinegar
¼ teaspoon black pepper
Salt to taste

1. Mix everything together. If using a blender the ginger and turmeric root will be obliterated into the mix, which is great but if you don't want this effect shake in a jar instead.

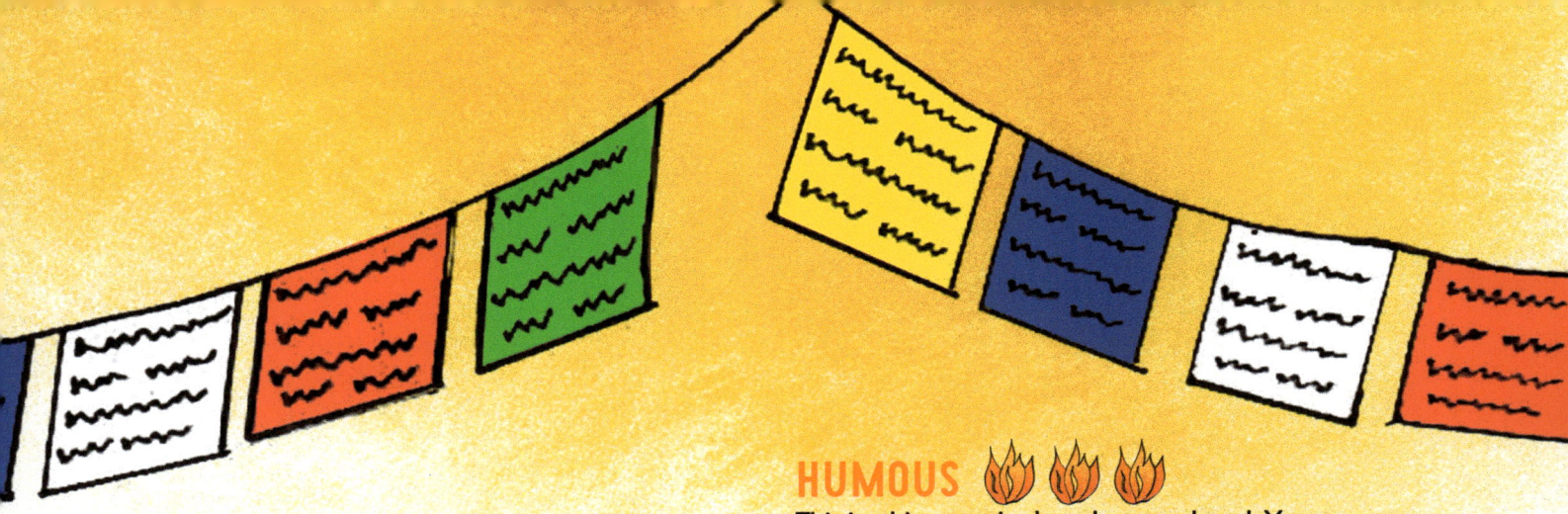

SPICY TIBETAN RAITA

I got this recipe from a monastery kitchen at Kopan in Nepal. I had it there with a masala omelette (see page 55) and it was so delicious I immediately went to the kitchen to ask what it was. As usual, the best things in life are so simple. They were delighted I loved it so much, and I am delighted to pass it onto you.

4 cups yoghurt (plant based is ok)
1 cucumber, grate and squeeze out the excess liquid
2 cups fresh coriander, finely chopped
1 cup fresh mint, finely chopped
1 or 2 green chillis (depending on how much heat you like)
1 teaspoon sea salt (it seems a lot but salt adds to the flavour in this quantity)

1. Put the yoghurt, salt, coriander, mint and chilli into a blender or bowl and mix or blend well together.

2. Stir in the grated cucumber and serve.

The best things in life are so simple

HUMOUS

This is a big quantity but always so loved. You can make this without a blender but it's a lot of mashing and mixing. Ideally use a blender.

Top tip: If you are cooking your own chickpeas put the garlic in and cook it with them, then use the cooled cooking water to make the initial mix.

3 cups dried (pre-cooked) chickpeas or two tins
1 tablespoon tahini
1 or 2 cloves of garlic (optional)
1 lemon, juiced
Olive oil, add as needed
Salt to taste
1 teaspoon ground paprika or ground cumin (optional)
1 handful of fresh herbs, parsley, coriander, basil and local seasonal herbs (optional)

1. Put the chickpeas, tahini, about ½ cup of water, the garlic (if using), lemon juice and any herbs or spices into a blender.

2. As you blend slowly pour in olive oil until you have a thick creamy consistency.

3. If using the optional herbs or spices add these after the initial mixture is nicely blended.

4. Lovely to serve in a big bowl with more olive oil poured over.

TAHINI CREAM
(blender only)

2 tablespoons tahini
1 lemon, juiced
1 clove garlic, roughly chopped
½ teaspoon cumin seeds

1. Mix everything together in a blender.

2. Slowly add water to your desired consistency (thick pouring cream).

BEETROOT RAITA

Raita is traditionally cucumber and yoghurt. I started playing around with combinations and this is a delicious and visually stunning alternative. You can also do this with 2 large carrots

1 large raw beetroot, peeled and grated
3 cups of yoghurt (plant or dairy yoghurt is fine)
1 teaspoon cumin seed
1 teaspoon caraway seed
1 teaspoon black mustard seed
1 tablespoon coconut oil or ghee

1. Melt the coconut oil or ghee in a small pan and sauté all the seeds until the mustard seeds begin to 'pop', a couple of minutes.

2. Add the grated beetroot and stir fry for 3 to 4 minutes, until it is softened.

3. Stir in the yoghurt, mix well and serve.

SLAW

½ a cabbage (red or white) finely shredded
1 sweet potato, grated
1 mooli radish, grated
2 cups cashew nuts, gently oven toasted
1 bunch fresh coriander, chopped

1. Mix together and toss with a dressing of your choice, turmeric dressing (page 76) is really lovely with this.

COURGETTE DIP
(blender only)

4 courgettes
1 head of garlic (omit if you have heat tendencies in the body)
1 lemon
Olive oil
1 teaspoon sea salt
1 teaspoon cumin seed

1. Preheat the oven to 200°C.

2. Chop the courgettes and smash the garlic cloves so the are all squidgy and oozing with their garlicky juices.

3. Chop the lemon into eight chunks.

4. Pile the lemons, courgettes and garlic into a baking tray and drizzle over a generous amount of olive oil.

5. Sprinkle the salt and the cumin seed over. Get in with your hands and rub the cumin, salt and olive oil well in with the garlic and courgettes.

6. Roast for 30 minutes or until the courgette are beginning to go nicely brown and sweet.

7. Leave to cool.

8. When completely cooled, put into a blender and whizz until it is creamy and smooth.

SOUPS.

SWEET POTATO SOUP.

1 stick celery, chopped
2 sweet potatoes, peeled and chopped (you can substitute pumpkin or squash)
1 carrot, chopped
1 inch ginger, chopped (optional, omit if you have heat tendencies in the body)
1 red chilli, chopped (optional, omit if you have heat tendencies in the body)
½ block of coconut cream or 1 tin coconut milk (or if you live somewhere with fresh coconut use this)
Churna spice mix for your dosha (see page 33)

1. Fry the celery in a little coconut oil until soft.

2. Add your churna spice mix, the sweet potato and carrot, plus the ginger and chilli (if using) and sauté together for a couple of minutes.

3. Add the coconut cream or milk and enough water to cover completely.

4. Simmer for 15 minutes until all the vegetables are cooked.

5. Blend and serve.

BEETROOT SOUP.

1 stick celery, chopped
2 fresh beetroots, peeled and chopped
1 parsnip, peeled and chopped
1 inch ginger, chopped (optional, omit if you have heat tendencies in the body)
1 red chilli, chopped (optional, omit if you have heat tendencies in the body)
1 teaspoon cumin seed
1 teaspoon caraway seed

1. Chop the celery and fry in a little coconut oil until soft.

2. Add the cumin seed, caraway seed, ginger and chill (if using), beetroot and parsnip and sauté together for a couple of minutes.

3. Add enough water to cover the vegetables.

4. Simmer for 30 minutes until all the vegetables are cooked.

5. Blend and serve.

HEARTY SOUP.

For hungry virtuous days, and using up left over vegetables

2 tins chickpeas or 3 cups of dried chickpeas soaked and cooked
1 courgette
2 sticks celery
1 clove garlic (optional, omit if you have heat tendencies in the body)
1 red chilli (optional, omit if you have heat tendencies in the body)
1 cup of fresh mixed herbs, parsley, coriander, oregano or 2 teaspoons of dried mixed herbs
1 teaspoon cumin seed
1 teaspoon fennel seed
1 teaspoon smoked (not hot) paprika
4 tablespoons tomato puree
Vegetables of choice, sweet or regular potato, greens, carrots.
Salt to taste

1. Chop the courgette and celery and fry in a little oil until soft.
2. Add the cumin seeds, fennel seeds, paprika, garlic and chilli (if using).
3. Add the chickpeas and stir.
4. Add enough water to cover the vegetables.
5. Bring to the boil and then simmer.
6. Stir in the tomato puree.
7. Chop up and add any other vegetables (except greens), simmer the whole lot until everything is cooked. The cooking time will vary depending on the vegetables you are using.
8. Add any fresh herbs and greens at the last minute. If using dried herbs add in five minutes before the end.

SOUP AND EXTRAS, A DELICIOUS AND SIMPLE MEAL IN A BOWL.

This came about by combining all kinds of random leftovers, and it's really yummy.

1. Make any soup as above.
2. Make a tahini dressing (see page 75).
3. Put cooked quinoa, rice or bulgar wheat into a soup bowl, ⅓ full.
4. Add soup on top and then the tahini dressing.

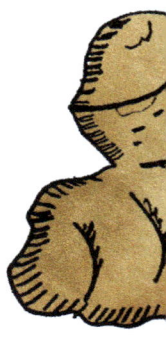

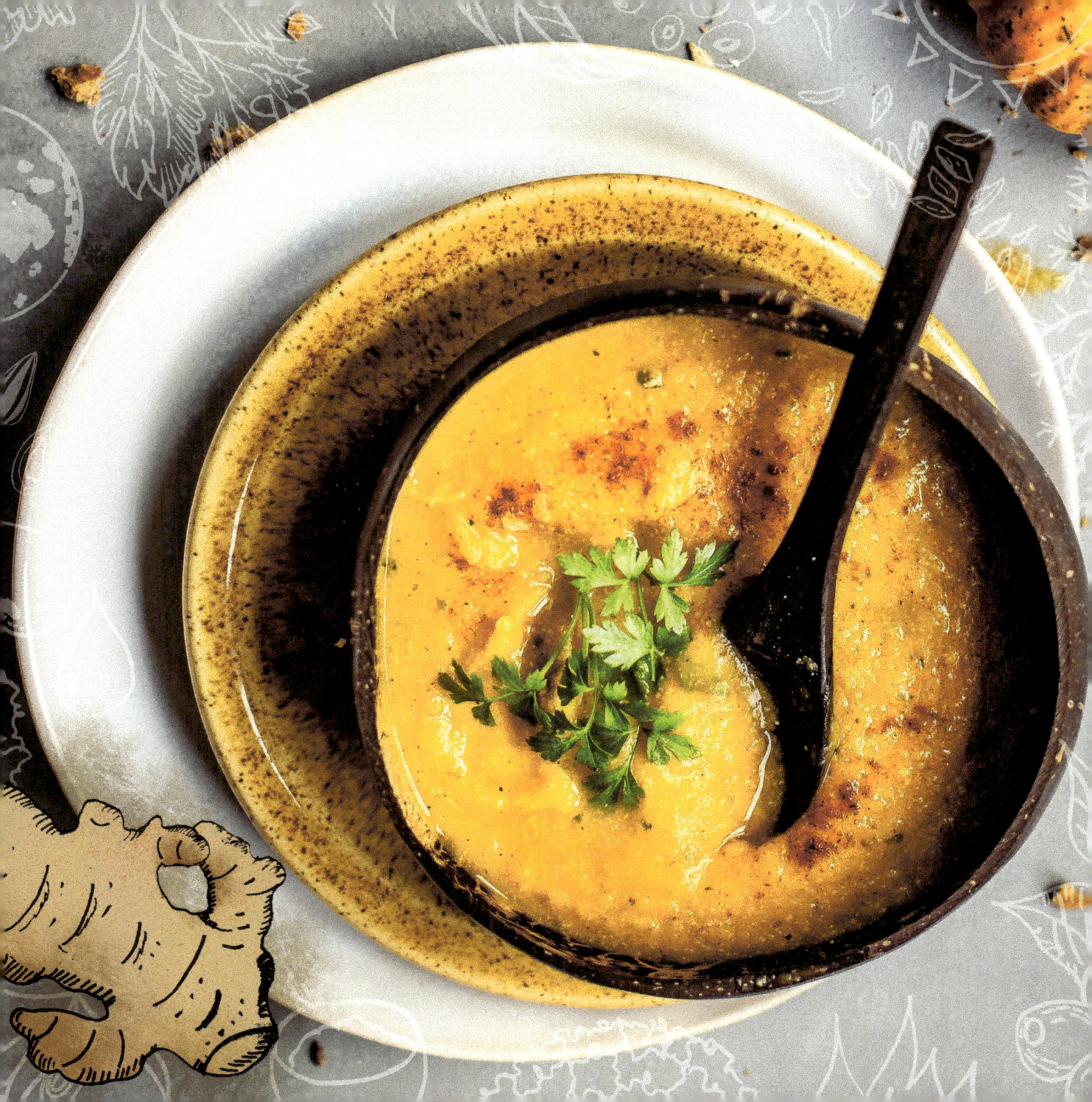

SWEET TREATS.

BANANA BREAD.

This recipe totally breaks the fruit rule and other guidelines, but it is delicious, especially with some almond butter. Flax eggs are the suggested option here. You can use regular eggs but they are not considered sattvic.

3 ripe bananas, peeled and quartered
10 medjool dates
3 tablespoons light tahini
2 teaspoons ground cinnamon
1 cup brown rice flour
4 flax eggs (1 flax egg = tablespoon ground flaxseed mixed with 3 tablespoons of water)
1 teaspoon bicarb soda

1. Preheat the oven to 175°C.
2. Grease and line a small loaf tin.
3. Place the bananas, dates, tahini and cinnamon into a food processor and blend until the mixture is smooth and well combined.
4. Add the rice flour, bicarb and flax eggs, mix to combine.
5. Pour the mixture into the prepared loaf tin.
6. Bake for 45 minutes until an inserted skewer comes out cleanly.
7. Leave the loaf in the tin to cool for five minutes before gently transferring to a cooling rack to cool completely.

OAT COOKIES.

You can be adventurous with your seeds, nuts and berries, try different things and see what you like best.

2 ½ cups rolled oats
½ cup wholewheat flour (or other flour of choice)
¾ cup coconut sugar
¼ cup sesame seeds
1 ½ teaspoons each of ground cinnamon and ginger
1 cup coconut oil, melted
½ cup water

1. Preheat your oven to 200°C.
2. Oil two baking sheets or use greaseproof paper.
3. Combine the dry ingredients in a bowl, add the oil and mix.
4. Stir in enough water to make a firm texture.
5. Take a ping-pong ball sized amount and shape into cookie shape (about 10cm in diameter).
6. Repeat with the remaining mixture.
7. Bake in oven for around 15 minutes until golden at edges.
8. Cool on a wire rack.

STEPHEN'S MUFFINS.

This recipe is from my teacher Stephen Brandon. Makes eight muffins.

1 ½ cups of plain flour
4 teaspoons baking powder
1 teaspoon cinnamon
¼ cup carob
½ cup molasses or rice syrup
3 tablespoons sunflower oil
½ cup plant milk of choice

1. Pre heat the oven to 180°C.

2. Mix all the ingredients together to make a batter.

3. Divide into eight greased muffin cases.

4. Bake for 15-20 minutes.

ALMOND COCONUT PRASAD.

Prasad is a traditional and devotional food offering to the divine. It is sometimes passed around in temples and at festivals and is also placed on an alter or shrine.

1 cup desiccated coconut
1 cup ground almonds
1 capful rosewater
1 teaspoon cardamom powder
2 tablespoons maple syrup (or more if it needs more to stick see how things go - it really is different each time!)

1. Place the coconut, almond and cardamom in a bowl and mix together.

2. Add the rosewater and maple syrup and mix until it sticks together when pressed firmly.

3. Roll into little balls. These taste beautifully exotic!

CHOCOLATE ALMOND DATES.

20 good juicy medjool dates
20 almonds, skin on
200g dark vegan chocolate

1. Line a baking tray with greaseproof paper.

2. Gently remove the stones from the dates. You will discover that what lies within is a perfectly shaped cavity where you can then place an almond. Do this with each date and almond in turn.

3. Melt the dark chocolate in a bowl over a simmering pan of water.

4. Dip each date in turn into the melted chocolate, ensuring it gets totally covered.

5. Place onto greaseproof paper tray and put into fridge to set. So delicious!

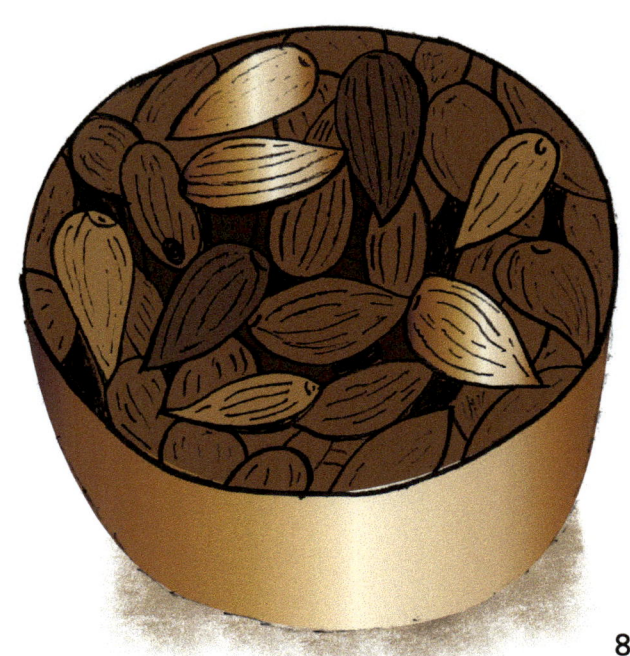

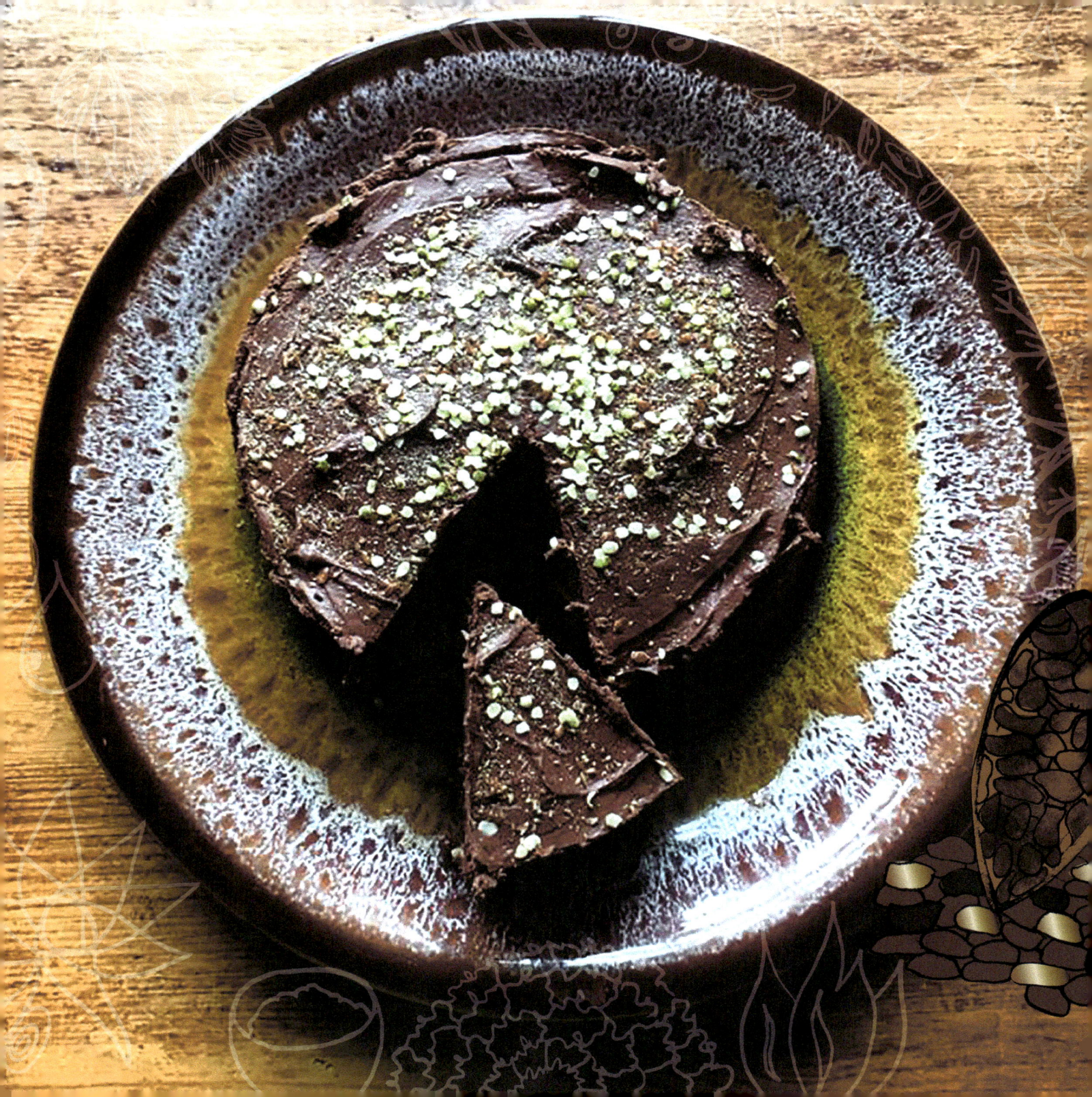

CHOCOLATE TORTE.

(Makes one large torte for up to 12 people).
This much-loved recipe has evolved over the years. I now make my own chocolate for this as well as using hemp and flaxseed for its nutritional benefits and you can optionally add some superfood powders too. Adapt it however you prefer. This is very rich so not much is required to satisfy a serious chocolate craving!

2 cups pitted medjool dates
1 cup walnuts
½ cup hempseed
½ cup flaxseed
3 tablespoons coconut oil (melted)
1 tablespoon ground cinnamon
75g cacao butter and 50g cacao powder
or 125g good quality vegan chocolate
Rice syrup to taste
1 pack of silken tofu
1 tablespoon maca powder (optional)
1 tablespoon ashwagandha powder (optional)

1. Blend the dates until they are very finely chopped.

2. Add the cinnamon, walnuts, seeds and coconut oil until you have a sticky stiff consistency.

3. Take this and press it firmly into an 24cm round tin, preferably one with springform sides or a loose bottom. Put this in the fridge to set whilst you put together the topping.

4. To make the chocolate melt the cacao butter (if it's a block chop it up a bit) in a bowl over a simmering pan of water, stir in the cacao powder and add rice syrup to taste. It is very bitter with no sweetener.

5. Alternatively melt regular chocolate over the simmering pan of water.

6. Blend the silken tofu until it is the consistency of thick cream.

7. Mix the two together to form a rich chocolatey gooey loveliness. Add in the maca and / or ashwagandha powder (if using) and blend these in thoroughly.

8. Pour the topping over the base and return to the fridge.

9. Serve in small slices with some cashew cream.

10. The topping can also be served on its own in a chocolate pot. It looks fabulous with some more hemp and flaxseeds sprinkled on top.

CASHEW CREAM.

This is a great and simple alternative to dairy cream.

1 cup cashew nuts
1 tablespoon rice or maple syrup
2 cups water
½ teaspoon cardamom powder (optional)

1. Soak the cashew nuts either overnight in cold water or in boiling water for one hour before you make the cream.

2. Drain and rinse the cashews.

3. Blend together the cashews, water, rice or maple syrup and cardamom powder (if using).

4. Check the consistency. The more water you add the thinner it will be. You can adapt for whatever you need from a thick cream to a thinner pouring consistency.

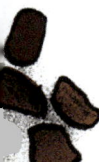

DRINKS AND SMOOTHIES.

You can make some of these drink and tea mixtures in advance and keep in a jar.

DIGESTIVE TEA.

1 teaspoon cumin seed
1 teaspoon coriander seed
1 teaspoon fennel seed

1. Place in a pan with two cups of water and gently simmer for ten minutes.
2. Strain and serve.

TURMERIC GINGER TEA.

2 inches fresh ginger root, grated
1 inch fresh turmeric root, grated

1. Add the ginger and turmeric to a pan with 500ml water.
2. Simmer for 20 minutes.
3. Strain and serve.
4. Lovely with a little honey stirred in at the last minute (do not cook or heat the honey). You can also keep the pulp and use another time. It's quite potent.

GOLDEN MILK.

This drink is comforting, sweet, grounding and nurturing. The turmeric is an incredible anti-inflammatory and anti-oxidant (and much more). The ashwagandha is renowned in ayurveda for being restorative and rejuvenative as well as relaxing. It promotes our vital ojas or life energy and is incredible for our immunity.

1 cup milk (any plant or dairy milk is fine)
½ teaspoon ground cinnamon
¼ teaspoon ground cardamom
1 pinch of ground nutmeg
1 teaspoon ashwagandha
½ teaspoon ground turmeric
Honey or maple syrup to taste (optional)

1. Pour the milk into a pan, leaving a small amount in the bottom of the cup.
2. Whilst the milk in the pan is heating add to the cup, the cinnamon, ashwagandha, cardamom, nutmeg, and turmeric.
3. Pour over the warm milk.
4. Add honey or maple syrup to taste.

BEETROOT ROSE LATTE.

When the heart is broken we can feel ungrounded, restless and maybe angry. These are pitta and vata traits. This gorgeous drink is super helpful in these tricky emotional times. The rose is healing for the heart and emotions plus cooling for pitta. The beetroot is sweet, grounding and nurturing for vata. The milk is soothing for both. The ashwagandha restores our ojas, our energy and vitality.

Perfect if you need to feel comforted, calmed and emotionally supported.

1 cup milk (any plant or dairy milk is fine)
1 capful rose water
1 teaspoon beetroot powder
1 teaspoon ashwagandha
Honey or maple syrup to taste (optional)

1. Pour the milk into a pan and heat gently, leaving a small amount in the bottom of the cup.
2. Whilst the milk in the plan is heating add to the cup the beetroot powder, ashwagandha, and rose water, stir into a paste.
3. Pour over the warm milk.
4. Add honey or maple syrup to taste.

SLEEP TEA.

1 teaspoon chamomile flowers
1 teaspoon lavender flowers
1 teaspoon valerian root

1. Place in a pan with two cups of water and gently simmer for ten minutes.
2. Strain and serve.

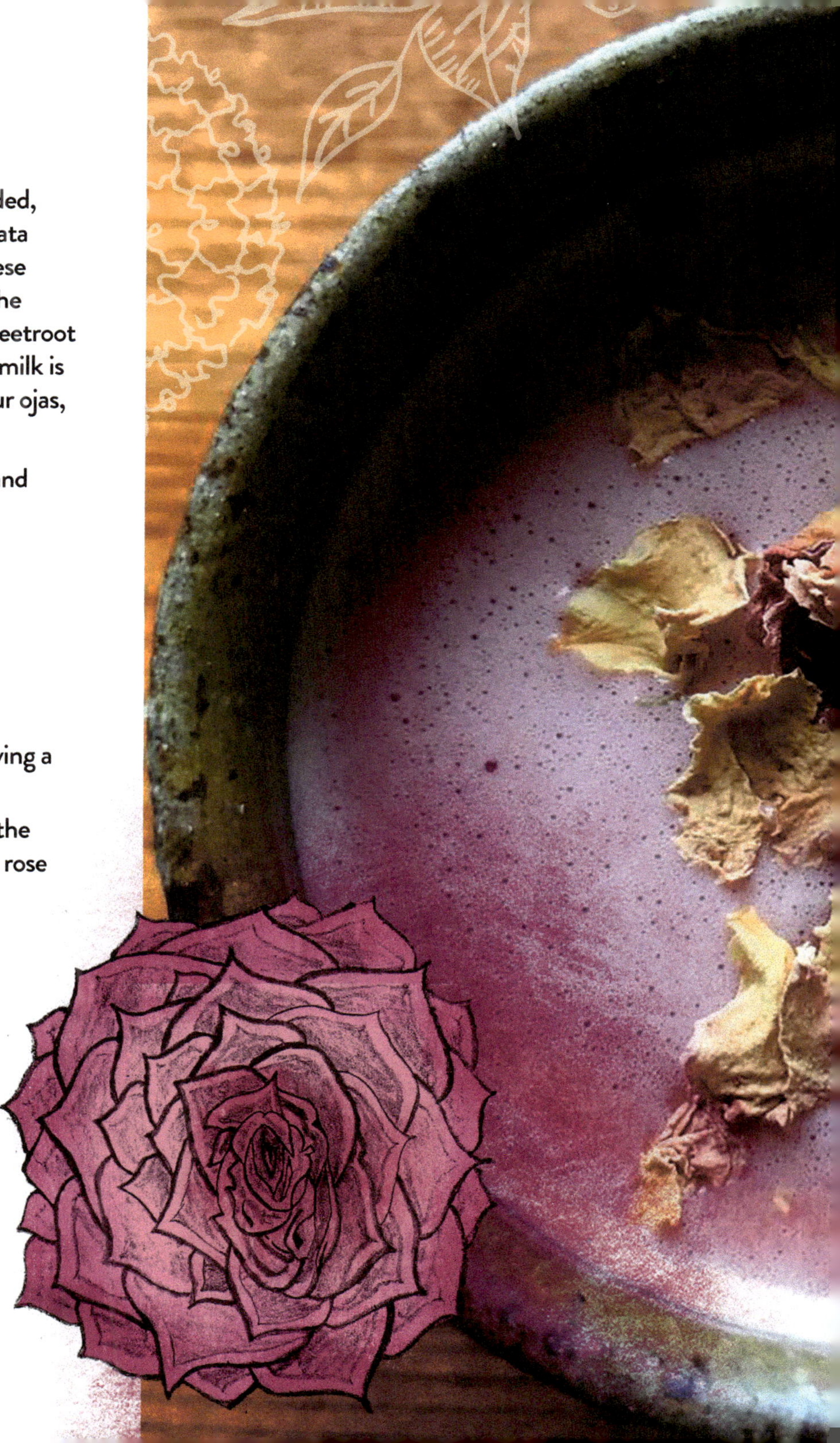

CHAI STYLE TEA.
(caffeine free herbal version)

Chai is the nectar of India. It is so sweet and delicious, it often comes in small clay cups, is already pre-sweetened and contains loads of sugar. There is nothing more magical than standing on the banks of the holy river Ganges in the slowly emerging dawn whilst sipping a hot cup of chai!

1 cinnamon stick
1 inch fresh ginger, grated
2 cloves
2 green cardamom pods
¼ teaspoon ground nutmeg
½ teaspoon of whole black peppercorns
500ml water

1. Put all the spices into a pan with 500ml of water and simmer for 20 minutes.
2. Strain and serve.

CHAI STYLE TEA.
(caffeine and milk version)

1 cinnamon stick
1 inch fresh ginger, grated
2 cloves
2 green cardamom pods
¼ teaspoon ground nutmeg
½ teaspoon of whole black peppercorns
1 dessertspoon black tea or 2 teabags
500ml milk, dairy, almond, oat or other choice

1. Put all the spices into a pan with 500ml of milk and simmer for 20 minutes.
2. Make a small 250ml pot of black tea.
3. Once the spices have simmered in the milk, strain the milk through a sieve into the black tea and mix together. You can add a sweetener here if you wish, traditionally this is served with lots of sugar!

LASSI.

Lassi is a traditional drink that is used in warm weather to cool the body. Therefore it is best avoided in cold damp weather. It is also seen mixed with all kinds of fruit and other ingredients. This recipe is for a simple traditional lassi drink. It is great for digestion and the health of the microbiome.

½ cup of yoghurt (full fat organic dairy is preferable but plant based will still be good)
½ cup water
1 teaspoon mixed of fennel, cumin and coriander seeds

1. Blend everything together pour and drink.

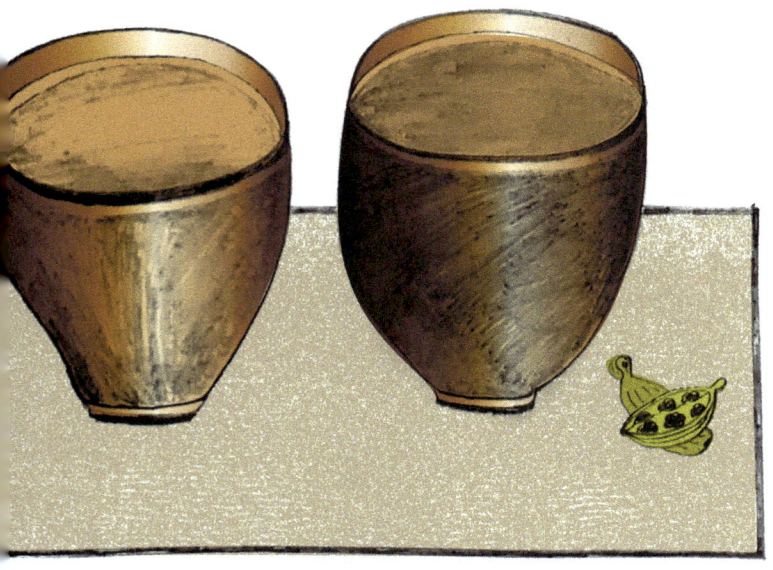

SMOOTHIES are not traditionally ayurvedic! However I have endeavoured to stick with ayurvedic principles when creating these. The same rules apply as for lassi, only during warm weather and to be avoided in cooler damper climates.

GREEN ENERGISING SMOOTHIE.

2-3 good sized kale leaves
Handful of spinach
1 stick celery
½ an avocado
1 teaspoon ashwagandha
1 teaspoon spirulina and wheatgrass powder mixed (or another greens mixture)
1 teaspoon moringa powder
1 teaspoon local honey
½ tablespoon hemp seeds
½ tablespoon flaxseeds
2 teaspoons hemp or black cumin seed oil
Water, add to desired consistency
(a thick shake)

1. Blend everything together pour and drink.

OM ANAM ANANDAM FOOD IS BLISS

OJAS (ENERGY AND VITALITY) SMOOTHIE.

I find when I am feeling depleted that this is a really rejuvenating pick me up.

1 cup oat, almond or other plant-based milk of choice (almond is traditionally more of an ojas rich food)
1 teaspoon ashwagandha
1 teaspoon ground turmeric
2 medjool dates
1 teaspoon local honey
1 tablespoon hemp seeds
1 tablespoon hemp or black cumin seed oil

1. Blend everything together pour and drink.

DECADENT AND DEFINITELY NOT AYURVEDIC SMOOTHIE.

300ml plant milk of choice (or use less and make a thicker consistency smoothie bowl to eat)
½ an avocado
1 small banana
1 teaspoon ashwagandha
2 medjool dates
2 teaspoons flaxseed
1 teaspoon hempseed
2 teaspoons cacao powder

1. Blend everything together pour and drink.

I hope you enjoy diving in and experimenting with all these beautiful food rituals!

You will find more recipes in the next chapter on cleansing.

BREATHE

Breathe in
breathe out
beginning and ending
birth, adulthood
death, regeneration
beginning and ending
forever evolving
learning to let go.

THE ISSUES ARE IN YOUR TISSUES

Life is a constant and consistent process of change. Humans in general find any kind of change, especially changes to their food, routine and lifestyle, incredibly challenging. And yet it is inevitable. By embracing becoming comfortable with change we can transition through life much more peacefully.

Once we have grown accustomed to a more supportive daily routine and begin to enjoy preparing simple, healthy, food we may want to explore a bit more. We can begin to introduce more seasonal awareness into the foods we are eating, to shop more locally, supporting the local economy and being more aware of sustainability in what we eat. We can become more aware of the changing seasons and of our own health needs at the different times of the year and of our own living organism of the bodymind.

The issues are in our tissues. Literally. This is why we place such importance and emphasis upon cleansing in ayurveda. The food we eat becomes our body tissues and cells, think about that for a moment. Even if we eat healthily today we may not have done in the past. In addition to the more physical stuff, the emotional reactions we have release chemicals into the body, leading to tension and diagnoses such as irritable bowel syndrome. If stress reactions and symptoms are common this can also create dis-ease. We literally hold on to everything in the body. These toxins, if left unchecked, lead to stagnation, inflammation and dis-ease, by cleansing them from the body we are massively helping to prevent disease. The process of cleansing helps to shift these toxins, called ama, on a cellular level. A cleanse can be a very simple process and is part of a way of living cyclically in tune with nature.

I use the term bodymind a lot. It's important to understand that the body and the mind are the same thing. Thoughts, feelings and emotions have an effect in the physical body in terms of our posture, breath, heartbeat, muscle tension, hormonal release, endorphins, adrenaline, digestion and much more.

If the mind is agitated the body is restless. If we are mentally exhausted the body will be tired.

The mind is the body.

The body is the mind.

So when we work with one we work with both, they are one.

BREATH.

We can introduce a regular breathing and mediation practice with this awareness in mind. The breath is said to contain everything we need to know about the cyclical nature of life. It teaches us about welcoming in whatever comes, how much tension can be created if we try to hold on and grasp, how delicious it feels if we can let go. And the stillness, the space of perfect peace at the end of each out breath. This is the gift of each and every breath cycle. Try sitting quietly noticing and reflecting on this.

The in-breath brings into the bodymind energy and oxygen, nourishing our tissues, cells and organs. It is a sense of renewal, of new beginnings and an opportunity to nourish ourselves. The in-breath is a new beginning, a rebirth, a new life opportunity, new energy and new experiences.

There is always (however brief) a small **pause at the end of each in-breath**, a tiny space just before we feel the trigger to breathe out. If we have a tendency to feel anxious we may breathe in deeper and hold the breath in more than usual. If we hold it too long, we may feel a kind of tension. This creates a feeling of increased tension in the bodymind. If you do get anxious it is worth noticing what your breath does and then see if a gentle awareness and shifting of this holding pattern helps. The pause at the end of the in-breath can potentially be a time of heightened energy, or an increase in tension, kind of like life! Our life experience, especially in adulthood, can be one of incredible energy and experience or it can feel very stressful.

Following this holding on state (and we hold on to so much in life), we begin to let go.

The out-breath has a real sense of release. Notice as you breathe out how it is not really possible to hold too much tension in the bodymind. The out-breath enables and supports us in letting go, physically, mentally, emotionally. The relief that comes with breathing out is noticeable. When we are uptight we automatically sigh, this is the bodymind's way of trying instinctively to release the held tension. In life we need to learn to let go, of people, places, things. Nothing is immortal or eternal, including us. This lifelong lesson, as we grasp on to life, to possessions, to relationships, is one that is so challenging, and yet it is the most incredibly powerful and healing practice we can begin to embrace. As we age, moving from adulthood into middle and older age, we need to learn to let go or we will suffer.

At the end of each and every single out-breath is a real gift. The gift of stillness. At the end of the out-breath there is a pause, a brief moment just before we have the trigger to breathe in again. In this moment there is nothing, there is simply a place of peace. After letting go there is stillness. Like a winter's morning and that special silence when snow has fallen, we can find a softness in this silence. At the end of each and every breath cycle we have this place of peace. This would not come if we did not let go. In order to be peaceful we must let go. This place of stillness allows for the life stage of death, then moves us into the stage of regeneration. However you view it, after we let go we do eventually die. This life cycle stage is guaranteed for everyone, so if we can learn to get used to the idea it will be helpful for us. Befriending the breath, particularly the out breath and the stillness of the pause helps us begin this process.

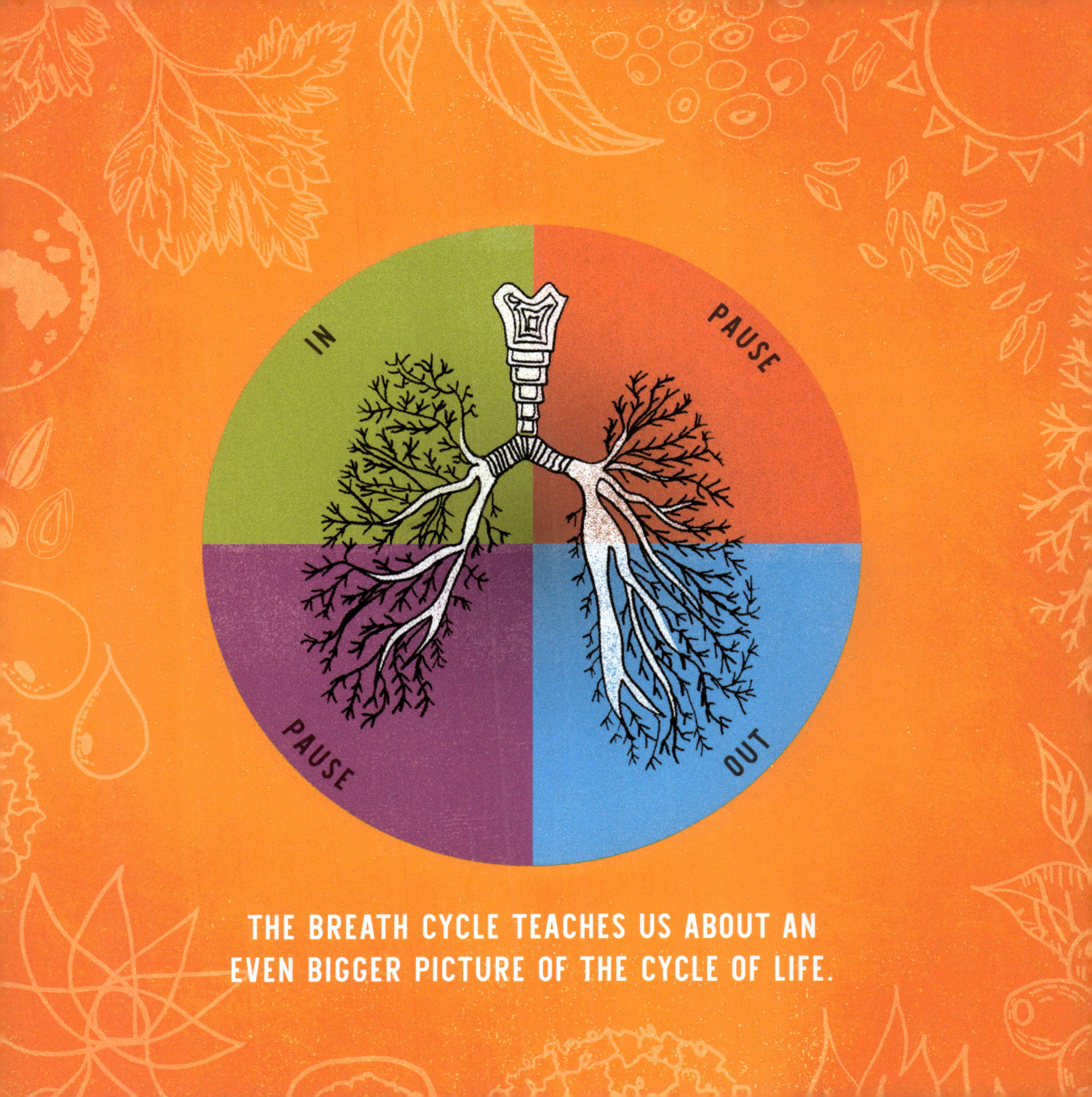

THE BREATH CYCLE TEACHES US ABOUT AN EVEN BIGGER PICTURE OF THE CYCLE OF LIFE.

After letting go there is stillness – a place of perfect peace.

These different stages of the breath can be used to help us to manage our emotions, to change how we feel. Because the breath reacts and responds to our emotions, we can change how we feel by working with this process and taking control of the breath.

Regeneration happens to all living biological organisms. Plants and trees especially, shedding seeds then regrowing, or perennial plants growing year after year. We don't know what happens to us when we die, but why shouldn't we also regenerate somehow? On the banks of the Ganges river in Benares, India, bodies are burned and then the ash joins the river, reuniting with the elements, returning to source, a complete cyclical process of regeneration,
returning us to the earth, water, fire, air and ether.

LETTING GO, GIVING STUFF UP, CLEANSING, A WAY OF REGENERATING OURSELVES.

Letting go may not be so final at first! As we journey through life we may wish to adopt healthier habits, to let go of unhelpful ways of behaving or not so healthy foods. This is not always easy. It may not be that everyone gives up everything, or that it is for the long term. We may do this as part of a cleanse, or we may do it for a few years and then find we need different foods as we age. Remember we are all unique and different.

WHAT KIND OF THINGS MAY WE WANT TO GIVE UP AND WHY?

Sugar: This is by far the most addictive food on the planet. The food industry have worked hard to put sugar into most prepackaged processed foods. Even those that appear healthy often contain a dose of this substance. Something can be labelled as low fat but may still be high in sugar. Fat has been promoted as the bad guy, when actually we need good fats in order to survive. Sugar is really the bad guy behind all of this and causes us to feel depleted and exhausted. We have sugar highs and bursts of energy followed by drops in our energy, and then we begin to continually crave this peaking and dipping effect in our bodymind. We crave the high. The remedy we then reach for instinctively is more sugar! It is incredibly hard to give up sugar, but it can be done.

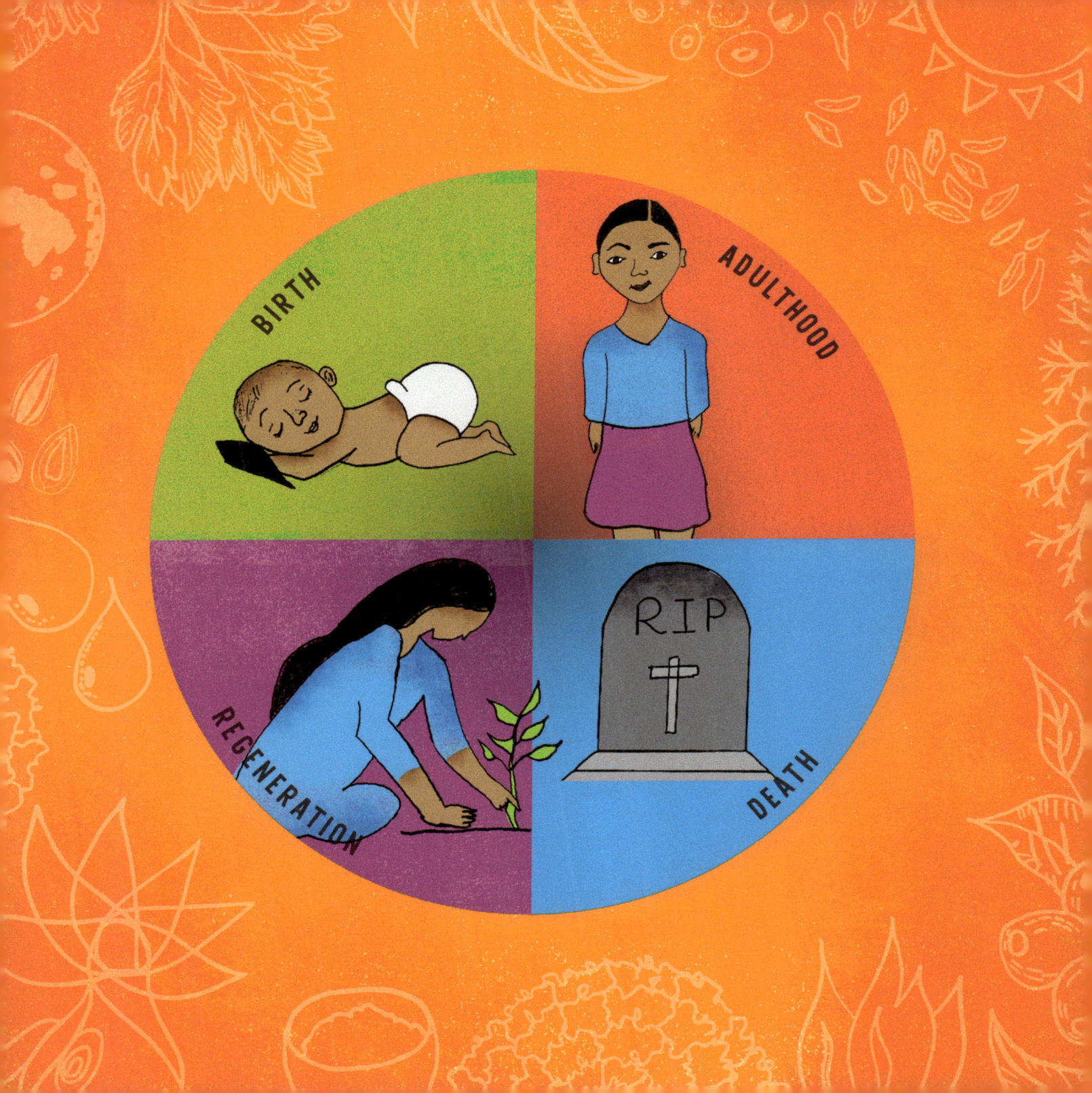

All recipes in this book are free of refined sugar. Substitutes are ok in moderation, such as rice syrup, date syrup, honey, coconut palm sugar and rapidura pure cane sugar. It's the refined white stuff and too much of any sugar that causes the trouble. As if this wasn't enough the sugar industry have found the exact level of sweetness that makes their product most addictive, and so every food you consume that contains this scientific equation makes you even more addicted. In my opinion the sugar industry are actually much worse than most drug dealers and use many of the same tactics.

Dairy: Any dairy product can create excess mucus in the body, especially if you are generally prone to this. Some people may benefit from having dairy in their diet. In excess too much dairy is not good, we don't need too much of it. A lot of the issues with dairy are that it comes from cows. Cows are often farmed with intensive farming methods, they may not even see a blade of grass. Calves are removed shortly after birth so the milk can be the taken for humans. The calves are often sold for veal.

A few years ago I lived for some months on a farm, as a lodger not a farmer! One weekend I heard the cows calling out constantly. This was because the calves had been removed for the milking to begin. The cry was so haunting and sad, truly that of a mother who had lost her child. The cow would have been stressed. So aside from the removal of the calf, the cow releases stress hormones into its system and into the milk. We then drink the milk. In addition there are often hormones that have been injected. I did eat dairy for many years. Now I do occasionally have natural yoghurt (curd) and ghee (clarified butter see page 103). It's important for me to ensure this comes from a sustainable and cruelty free source. In ethical sustainable farming the cow keeps the calf. The calf takes what milk it needs from its mother and then the farmer takes a little milk afterwards. There are places where this milk can be sourced, you just need to research a bit to find them.

Alcohol: If alcohol were invented now it would not be legal. In addition, it contains sugar (see above). The human condition that is created by our life experience can make us want to escape reality, and alcohol is a fine, readily available, very socially acceptable and effective remedy to our reality. Alcohol, and it is the same with any other consciousness altering substance, alters our perception of reality. It changes how we feel, think and function. I am not saying alcohol is evil, but we have to be aware that it changes who we are on some level. For some it is a really problematic issue. It can also be highly addictive. Stopping alcohol suddenly if you drink on a daily basis may be risky and you should seek professional advice if you intend to do this.

Caffeine: In a smiler way to sugar caffeine gives us energy peaks and dips. If consumed regularly it can be highly addictive. Granted, some people seem to be much more sensitive to caffeine than others. I'm very aware as I am writing this that I want to say that it's not so bad and, and that's because I am a total caffeine addict – or at least I was when I was drinking coffee. So you see how it works? We totally seek to justify our behaviours.

An excess of caffeine, and everyone's level of what they can tolerate is different, can cause heightened anxiety, sleep disturbances, digestive issues, high blood pressure (due to its stimulatory effect) and an increased heart rate. If we drink it regularly, we may find that when we stop we get a caffeine withdrawal headache and feel depleted in energy. It also drastically affects our sleep - even if we do only drink it before midday we can grossly underestimate what an impact caffeine has on our whole system.

Meat and animal products: There are several reasons not to eat animal products (this includes, meat, fish and eggs). A lot of the reasons are ethical, the intensive factory farming and general poor animal welfare and conditions are not only cruel for the animal, but the meat is then full of stress hormones and not healthy. In addition animal products are a lot harder for our digestive system to process. If you eat meat you may have experienced excess heat or sweating afterwards as the body is trying to break it down. In the past when we were hunter gatherers we would have eaten meat but much less often and the vast majority of our food would have been plant based. As with dairy it may be that you don't eat meat for some years then as you begin to age you feel your body needs it occasionally.

One thing I have definitely learned is never say never. **Our bodymind is continually changing and evolving. Years ago I ate a lot of dairy, then I was totally vegan, now I eat it very occasionally. These days sometimes, maybe once a month, I eat oily fish. I no longer drink coffee yet I used to have a whole cafetière full to the brim every morning. We are, all of us, always a work in progress.**

How do we give stuff up?
It's not easy to let go of these foods and habits that are often ingrained in our psyche and society. If we want to see friends, go out and about, be sociable, often food and routine are factors. If we stop drinking alcohol or decide we want to be in bed by 9.30pm, then we can be seen as 'weird'. We crave a feeling of belonging, of wanting to feel included and so we are reluctant to give up what enables us to feel part of everything. This is why it isn't straight forward or simple. This is why we might stop, for example coffee, for a while and then have it again. This applies to any kind of behavioural change. We stop, start, stop, start for a bit. Then we may stop completely. It is a good idea not to be too hard on yourself. It can be helpful to have an 80/20 rule. So you are not saying never again, you are saying most of the time. And only do it if you feel it is helpful for you. This is not meant as a punishment, it is intended to help you enhance your health and feel the best version of you that you can possibly be.

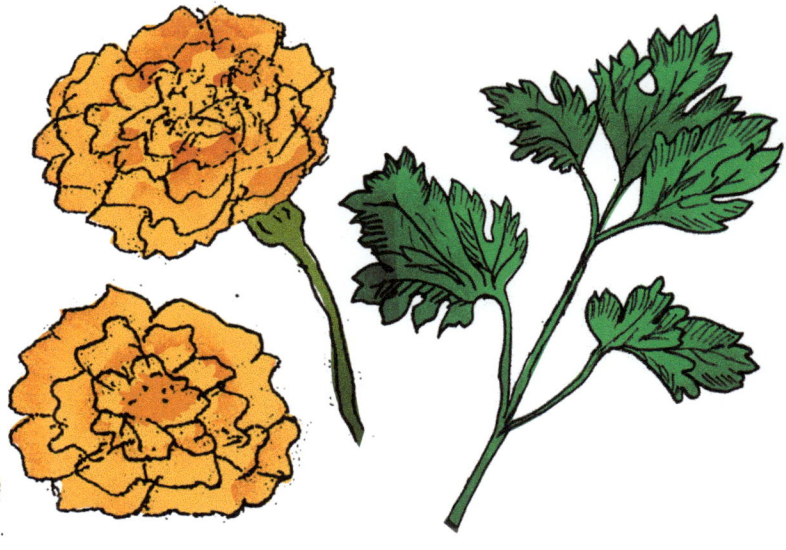

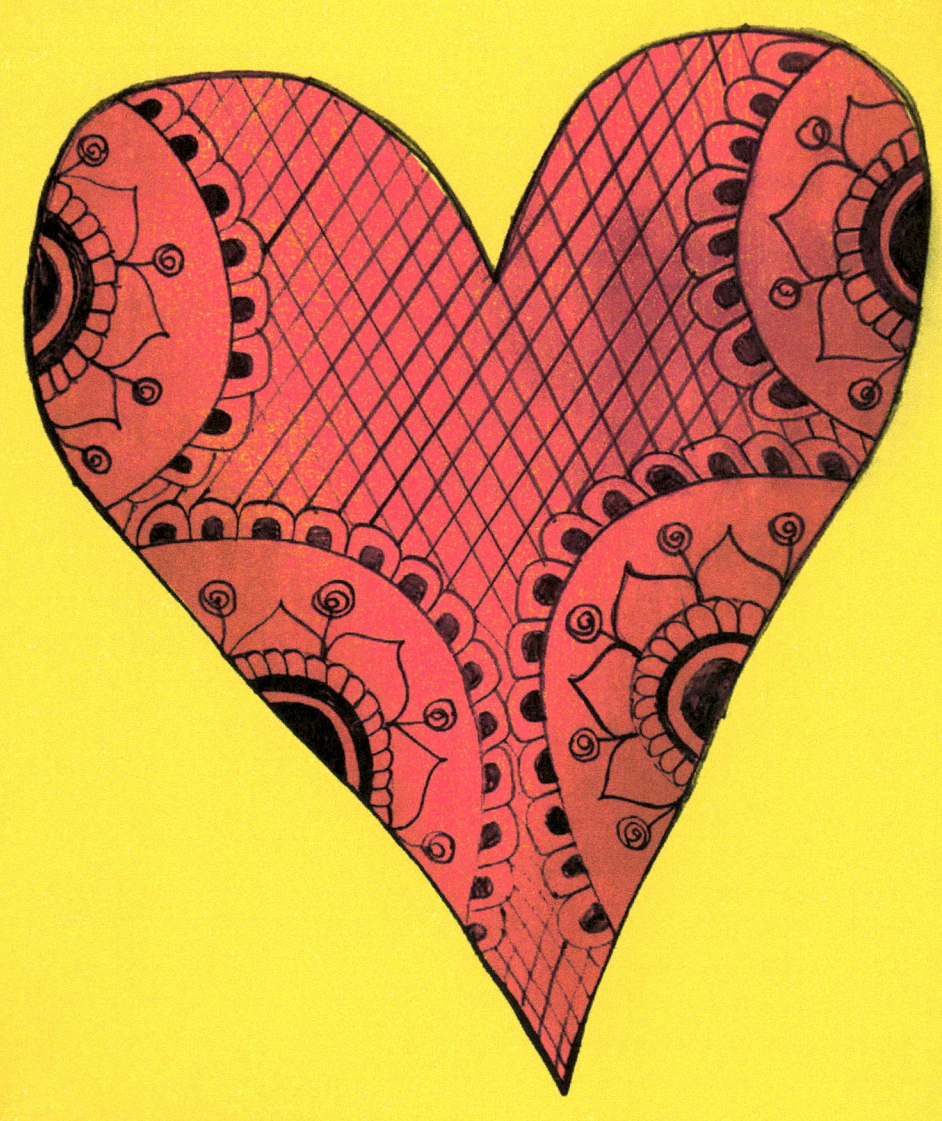

Food is emotional. As children growing up our family or carers often have specific behaviours, scenarios, rituals and rules around food, these can be helpful or unhelpful. This experience can shape how we feel and manage food for our whole lifetime. As a child I remember that it was rare for my parents to go out in the evening. When they did very occasionally they would often return late evening and have cheese and biscuits. I was allowed to get back out of bed and join them. Later in life I had a serious cheese addiction, and I still continued to enjoy cheese and biscuits as a 'treat'. It took me a lot of inner reflection to link these things together. My parents split when I was ten and so the feeling I got when I treated myself to this childhood delight, even as an adult, was comforting and gave me that much needed sense of security and belonging. It was only when I began to get mucus related chest problems in my early 30s that I tried stopping cheese. I never thought it was possible for me to stop! However I have not had any health issues since, and now I truly don't even miss it. It really is worth noticing the emotional impact of old favourites upon you, and perhaps take some time to reflect on what this may really be about.

FASTING AND CLEANSING

Fasting and cleansing have many physical and health benefits, and also help us regenerate the bodymind. They can be practiced as part of your regular routine. A suggestion is to do a longer (three days to one week) cleanse twice a year and a one day cleanse each month on the new moon. Hence cleansing becomes part of this cyclical process which we can find ourselves leaning into more and more.

A fast can be really simple. It can be missing supper, so you don't eat from lunchtime until the following breakfast time, or miss breakfast so you don't eat from supper until the following lunch time, or do twenty four hours from one lunchtime until the next. After 16 hours with no food the body automatically begins to heal itself. It is very simple and powerful. In general this method of fasting can help you to lose weight and body fat, if this is what your goal is. It also boosts your metabolic rate, so you process and utilise the energy from your food more effectively. There is an improvement in heart health as you reduce the level of 'bad' cholesterol in your blood. Studies have also shown that fasting helps regulate your blood sugar and hence helps prevent diabetes. Because of all these benefits regular fasting, even for just 16 hours, helps us live longer and feel healthier in general. If we feel healthy we feel happier and we tend, on the whole, to have a better quality of life. This method of fasting can be done once or twice a week.

A cleanse does include eating but is usually focused around a specific diet or type of food. I hate to use the word diet, this is not a 'diet' in the traditional or usual sense, it is a way of being and an integral part of your lifestyle. There is an absolute multitude of cleansing retreats, practices, trends and recommendations on offer. The information I am sharing with you in the next few pages is based on a traditional ayurvedic method. It is generally done twice a year at a change of season depending on the climate. In UK this would usually be in the spring and autumn.

It is helpful when cleansing, and if possible even if doing a short fast, to be quieter. During this time energy levels may feel lowered. It may be helpful to plan some time away from being online, watching TV, being on the phone and away from a hectic schedule. If you can a massage will aid the resetting process. Therefore this is time you set aside just for you, to take especially good care of yourself. To let go for a while, to settle into the stillness and to regenerate.

EATING MINDFULLY

Generally, in ordinary everyday life, when we eat we can be preoccupied with other things. Eating at the desk is common if we don't have a long lunch break, eating watching TV in the evenings to 'switch off'. If we don't focus on our food whilst we are eating this may affect our ability to digest our food (see 'a word about digestion' on page 50). So especially when cleansing, please ensure you are able to take the time to eat slowly and mindfully and don't do anything else at the same time. The process of eating, digesting and absorbing all of the nutritious content from the food you have lovingly prepared for yourself is miraculous. Take some time to appreciate this.

BLESSING THE FOOD DURING CLEANSE

For the duration of the cleanse you may wish to bless your food after you have prepared it and before you eat. You can do this however you wish. It may be that you sit silently and really look at the food before eating and appreciate all the effort to bring this to the plate in front of you. Or you may wish to use a more formal blessing such as saying Om Anam Anandam, meaning food is bliss. This isn't essential but it may enhance your cleanse experience and help you feel fully focused.

A SIMPLE SUGGESTED CLEANSE

This cleanse can be done from between three days to one week. It is possible to do it for longer, but good to then have the support of an ayurvedic practitioner or therapist. It is also very beneficial to do this for just one day if that's all that you are able manage.

This cleanse is very simple. It is a monodiet (so just one food) of kitchari. Kitchari is a traditional ayurvedic healing food.

If this feels a bit much you could have stewed apple for breakfast (See breakfast recipes page 54) and / or a simple vegetable soup for supper.

This cleanse is all done within the parameters of the daily routine I have already described, (page 22) so breakfast by 8:30am, lunch between 12noon and 2pm, with the most food at this time, and supper by 7pm at the very latest.

Kitchari (pronounced kit-char-ee) is the traditional cleansing food of ayurveda. It is a combination of split moong lentils and white basmati rice with plenty of spices, depending on your constitution. Moong daal are small yellow lentils. They can get confused sometimes with yellow split peas, which are bigger. Often if you are in the supermarket they aren't with the other dried pulses, you'll find them in 'world foods.' Or order them online. Make sure you get the right thing.

It is important to use white rice because it is easier to digest. The combination of rice and moong dal provides all the amino acids needed to form a complete protein. Eaten on their own, each of these foods is missing one or more of the essential amino acids that our bodies are not able to make on their own. However, together they make the magic happen! The protein content of kitchari supports stable blood sugar levels so energy and mental clarity are balanced during the cleansing process.

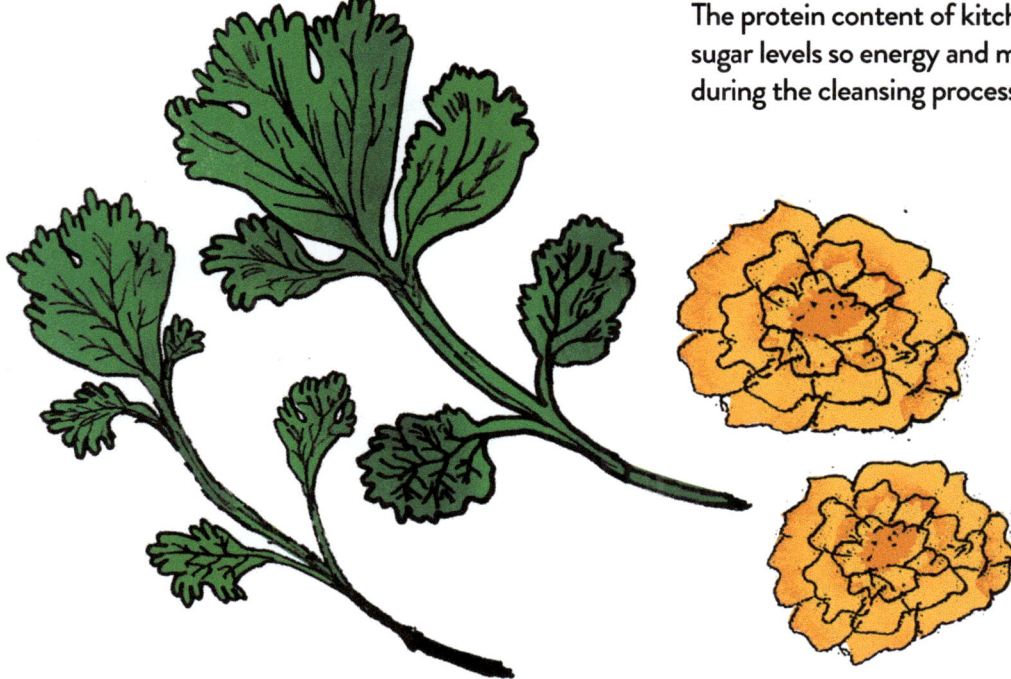

KITCHARI.

This recipe makes a good size portion for two people.

1 cup yellow moong dal
½ cup white basmati rice
2 tablespoons ghee (or coconut oil)
½ teaspoon ground coriander
½ teaspoon cumin seed
½ teaspoon fennel seed
1 teaspoon turmeric
½ teaspoon hing (asafoetida)
5 cups of water
½ teaspoon ground ginger (optional)
½ teaspoon black mustard seed (optional)
1 tablespoon fresh chopped herbs, coriander and parsley (optional)
Salt and pepper to taste
2–5 cups of chopped seasonal vegetables. In spring or warmer weather greens are lovely to use as they're so light and cleansing after the heaviness of winter. In autumn or cooler weather root vegetables feel very nurturing and grounding after the lightness and brightness of summer.

1. Rinse the mung dal and rice until the water runs clear.

2. Measure out all the dried spices.

3. Heat the ghee or oil in a large pot.

4. Add all the spices and sauté together on a medium heat for a minute or so until fragrant.

5. Stir in the mung dal and rice.

6. Add five cups of water and bring to the boil, then reduce to a simmer with the lid on.

7. Cook for at least 40 minutes, or until the dal and rice are completely soft (easily squashed between finger and thumb), the kitchari has a porridge-like consistency with the ghee or oil risen to the top, add more water if necessary.

8. Add vegetables at the appropriate time for them to cook in the kitchari, or cook them separately and stir in.

9. Adjust the seasoning and garnish with fresh chopped herbs if you like.

Slow cooker option

1. Rinse the moong daal and rice together in a sieve until the water runs clear

2. Measure out all the spices.

3. Heat the ghee or oil in a large pot.

4. Add all the spices and sauté together on a medium heat for a minute until fragrant.

5. Stir in the moong daal and rice.

6. Add to the slow cooker with five cups of water.

7. Heat on medium for 4-5 hours.

8. Add seasonable vegetables at an appropriate time for them to cook or cook them separately and stir in.

9. Once cooked adjust the seasoning and garnish with fresh herbs if you like.

GHEE, GOLDEN NECTAR!

Ghee (clarified butter) is revered in ayurveda for its healing and medicinal qualities. It is used in medicines and in everyday cooking. The benefits are many and include, healthy digestion, enhancing absorption of nutrients from food and aiding the healing qualities of herbs, boosting the microbiome and body's immune functioning, helping eliminate toxins, nourishing the brain and nervous system, it is also incredibly anti-inflammatory. Ghee may sometimes be more easily tolerated by those who are dairy intolerant because most of the lactose and milk fats are removed. Having been vegan for many years I was always reluctant to embrace this product, but now I understand a lot more about its benefits I include it as part of my regular diet.

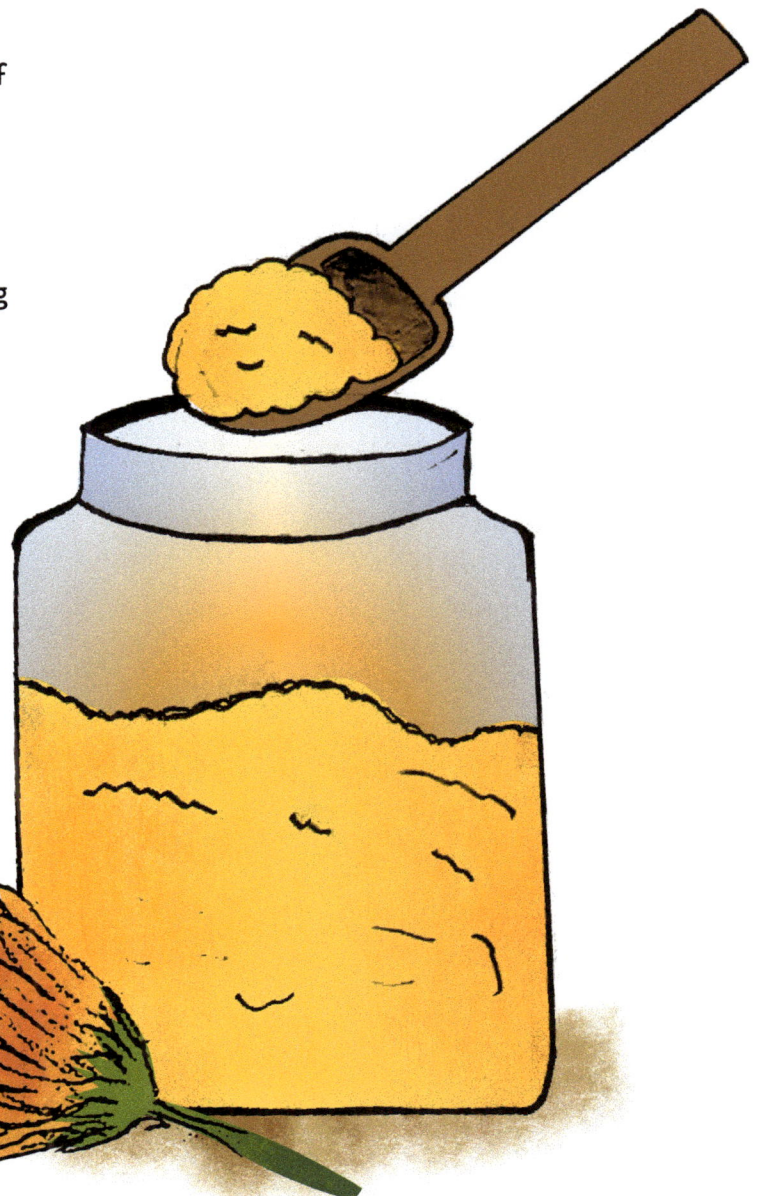

The following are suggestions and a nice addition to the cleanse process. Use them as described in the sections below as part of your cleanse routine. If in doubt please consult a practitioner.

Triphala

This ayurvedic herbal preparation (which means and contains) three fruits, haritaki, bibhitaki and amalaki, is an herbal concoction that has been used for thousands of years. Traditionally it is used as a digestive system tonic. Triphala promotes digestive regularity. The importance of this cannot be understated, especially for those who suffer from irregular elimination and other forms of bowel disease. Triphala can be in a tablet form or powder. Traditionally the powder was always preferred because the taste is considered an important part of the healing process. (See the suppliers information on page 139 for where to buy this).

During your cleanse: If using powder, *one teaspoon in a glass of warm water at night before bed is ideal, or if tablets then two tablets.* The taste can be strong so do drink it down quickly and then perhaps have a herbal tea afterwards. Do not use triphala in large doses as it can cause loose stools.

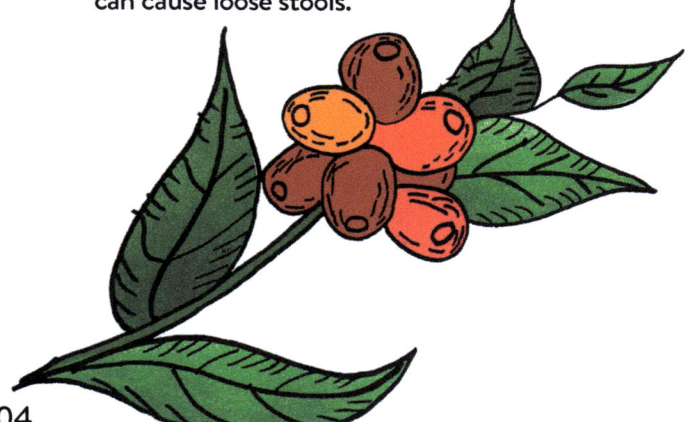

REJUVENATING TONIC.

This is fabulous if you are feeling depleted. Makes ½ a litre. Take one tablespoon twice a day.

1 large beetroot, chopped
A good handful (with gloves) of nettle leaves (dried or fresh)
1 tablespoon ashwagandha
1 tablespoon ground cinnamon
6 tablespoons molasses
500ml water

1. Put the beetroot and nettles into a pan with 500ml water, simmer for 30 minutes.

2. Strain the liquid into a bowl using a sieve.

3. Stir the ashwagandha, cinnamon and molasses into the liquid.

4. Allow to cool then bottle and store at room temperature.

The ashwagandha is a great energy boost and the cinnamon with the sweet molasses (also rich in iron) is super grounding for excess vata. Beetroot aids blood oxygen uptake, supports healthy digestion, is anti-inflammatory. Nettles are also anti-inflammatory, contain loads of nutrients for immunity and healing, both are high in iron so great if you're feeling run down and in need of a boost.

Ashwagandha

One of the most powerful ayurvedic herbs, ashwagandha is a root that has been used since ancient times for a wide variety of conditions and is most well-known for its restorative benefits. Ashwagandha means 'the smell of a horse', indicating that the herb imparts the vigour and strength of a stallion. It has traditionally been prescribed to help people strengthen their immune system after an illness. More recently this incredible plant has been evidenced as effective in treatment and management of post-viral fatigue and related conditions.

HEALING BROTH.

Good to have in the evening.

2 carrots, chopped or 1 sweet potato, cubed
1 stalk of celery, roughly chopped
1 onion, sliced
1 cup parsley, finely chopped
1 bulb garlic
1 inch ginger root
1 inch turmeric root
4 cups water

1. Place all the ingredients in a pot and bring to a gentle boil.

2. Turn the heat down low and allow to simmer for about an hour.

3. Strain through a colander and sip for a mineral rich, healing and restorative broth or leave the veggies in to enjoy as a light healing soup.

FIRE CIDER.

This needs to be made four to six weeks in advance. Makes ½ a litre.

2-4 cloves garlic, peeled and diced
½ onion, peeled and diced
3 inches ginger, peeled and diced
3 inches turmeric root, peeled and diced or 2 teaspoons dried
2 inches horseradish root, peeled and diced
1 red chilli, sliced
1 lemon, squeezed and quartered
2-4 sprigs rosemary
2-4 sprigs thyme
1 teaspoon black peppercorns
1 teaspoon coriander seeds
Raw unfiltered apple cider vinegar, enough to cover

1. Add all ingredients to a wide neck bottle or a jar.

2. Pour in the apple cider vinegar until it covers the ingredients and stir well.

3. Leave in a cool, dark place for four to six weeks, shaking occasionally.

4. Strain through a sieve into a clean bottle or jar and store in a cool dark place. This lasts several months.

Great for excess kapha (mucus and stagnant energy), and for winter cold and flu prevention. Take two to three teaspoons daily.

Caution if you have high pitta (fire/heat) and vata (air/movement), limit it to smaller amounts - one teaspoon daily only before 1pm

SWEET RICE.

This is a lovely option to 'break' your cleanse with on the last evening or morning. It is nurturing, grounding and sweet.

½ cup white basmati rice
3 cups boiling water
1 tablespoon black raisins
½ teaspoon ground cardamom
½ teaspoon ground cinnamon
¼ teaspoon ground ginger,
A small sprinkle of grated nutmeg
1 teaspoon turmeric powder
Twist of black pepper
Local honey or maple syrup to taste

1. Place the rice in a large pan with the water and bring to a gentle simmer.

2. Add water if the rice starts to look stodgy. Keep adding water to keep it simmering for around three hours. You can do this in two parts you can simmer for one or two hours, then another hour before serving. It will disintegrate into a porridge constancy. You do not need to add any milk, it will create its own sweet milky liquid as it cooks.

3. One hour before you are ready to eat add one tablespoon of black raisins.

4. 30 minutes before you are ready to eat add the ground spices. Lovingly stir in these spices.

5. Continue to allow it to gently simmer, adding more liquid if you need to.

6. When ready to eat stir in maple syrup or honey to taste, do not heat the honey just stir it in.

Slow cooker option.

1. Put the rice and water into the slow cooker on a medium heat for four to five hours.

2. Add more water if it begins to look stodgy.

3. Add the black raisins one hour before eating.

4. Stir in the spices 30 minutes before serving.

5. Add the honey or maple syrup at the very end.

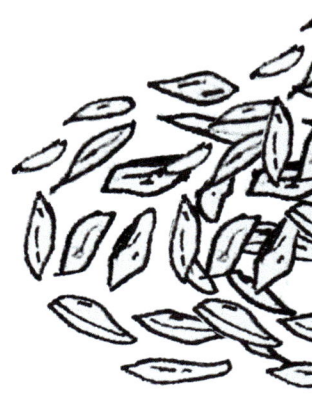

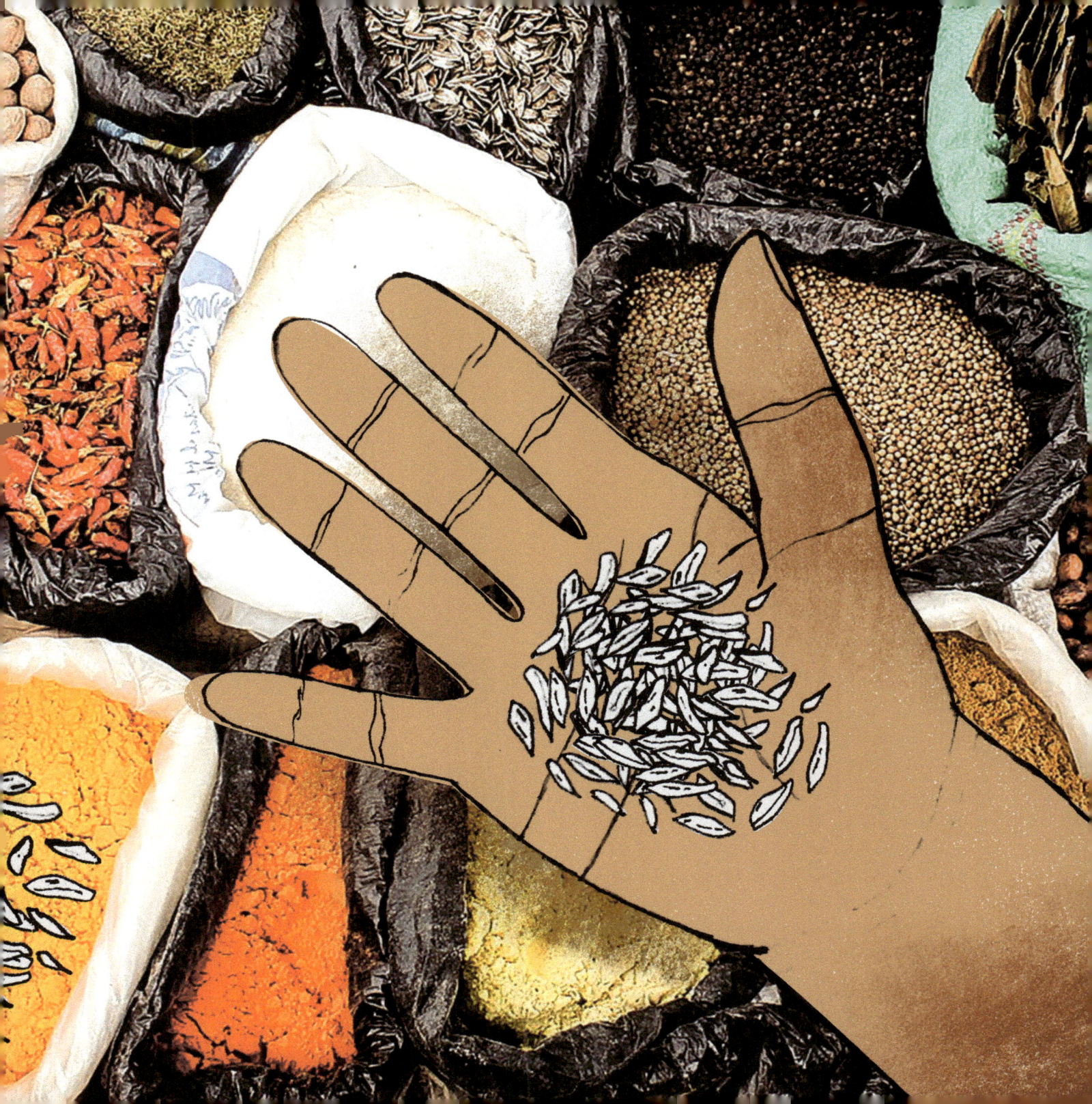

NEW MOON ONE DAY CLEANSE.

On page 44, I talked about a cleanse for one day each month near to the time of the new moon. This is a suggestion of how that day might look.

1. Fast until lunchtime, so no food but do enjoy some hot water and lemon or herbal tea.
2. Practice cleansing breathing and self-massage (see page 24).
3. Enjoy gentle and nurturing physical activity, such as restorative yoga.
4. Have kitchari for lunch.
5. In the afternoon walk in nature if possible. Bear in mind that your energy levels may be low so be mindful of how far you plan to walk.
6. Prepare things for the new moon bath and ritual in the evening (see page 44).
7. Have a light supper of soup or sweet rice.
8. Perform your chosen new moon ritual.
9. Enjoy your new moon bath.
10. Have some triphala before you go to bed followed by a herbal tea.

After your cleanse

Whatever length of cleanse you have chosen to enjoy it is good to plan for what happens next. Your body will be a bit more sensitive to any foods you have stopped for a while, even after one day you will notice a difference. We can become super sensitive to things we may have not noticed affected us before because we have purified the bodymind system.

If you have stopped things like sugar and caffeine you may not want to return to these. It is worth doing some planning to consider how you are going to go about your daily routine so you don't inadvertently slip back into old habits. For example, if you always had sugar in your tea at a particular place, when you visit that place again this urge may come back. It is important to know and understand so that we don't trip ourselves up in this way. If you are planning on changing your food and routine completely this is totally achievable, depending on how things were before, it's important to understand this can be a massive undertaking.

Eating out. Often this can be late in the evening. Occasionally this is ok but you will feel the difference if you have become used to eating earlier. Eat before you go out then join people to see them and enjoy their company, but not for food. This sounds odd I know but it does help and other people do get used to it!

Be aware of where you are going. Some venues definitely don't serve food that will be ok for your body. Point blank avoid these places. Do not compromise on your health and well-being. Find places that serve food you can feel ok about eating. It is your body, your health and only you can decide to do this.

Introduce other foods back in slowly. For example if you have stopped dairy have a very occasional bit of cheese. By occasional I mean once or twice a month and in moderation. Be aware of the seasonal adaptations you can make. Remember cheese is mucus forming so you may wish to avoid it in cooler weather but can have it a bit more in warm weather.

Go slowly and gently. Don't beat yourself up if you do revert back to old habits. Get up the following day and begin again. Remember that this is a gradual cyclical process.

Plan a regular cleanse. One day a month at new moon, twice a year for a longer cleanse. Build this into your lifestyle. Your bodymind will really thank you for it in the long term.

SUKKAH AND DUKKA

The general state that we exist in a lot of the time is dukkha. This means suffering. We may not be visibly wounded or injured, but a lot of our behaviour is geared toward avoiding or not feeling, and this in itself causes suffering.

Sukkha mean sweet spot, happiness, feeling that you are in a good space which is full and positive. Being in the space of sukkha is sattvic and allows genuine authentic happiness to arise. We can only achieve this state for ourselves. We cannot rely on external factors or other people to make us happy.

If our life has structure, if the bodymind has an inner strength and flexibility, if we feel we have a sense of purpose, then we are more likely to experience this state of sukkha. In order to reach this we need to care for the body with appropriate food and exercise, with physical, emotional and psychological care of ourselves. We need to become architects of our own destiny.

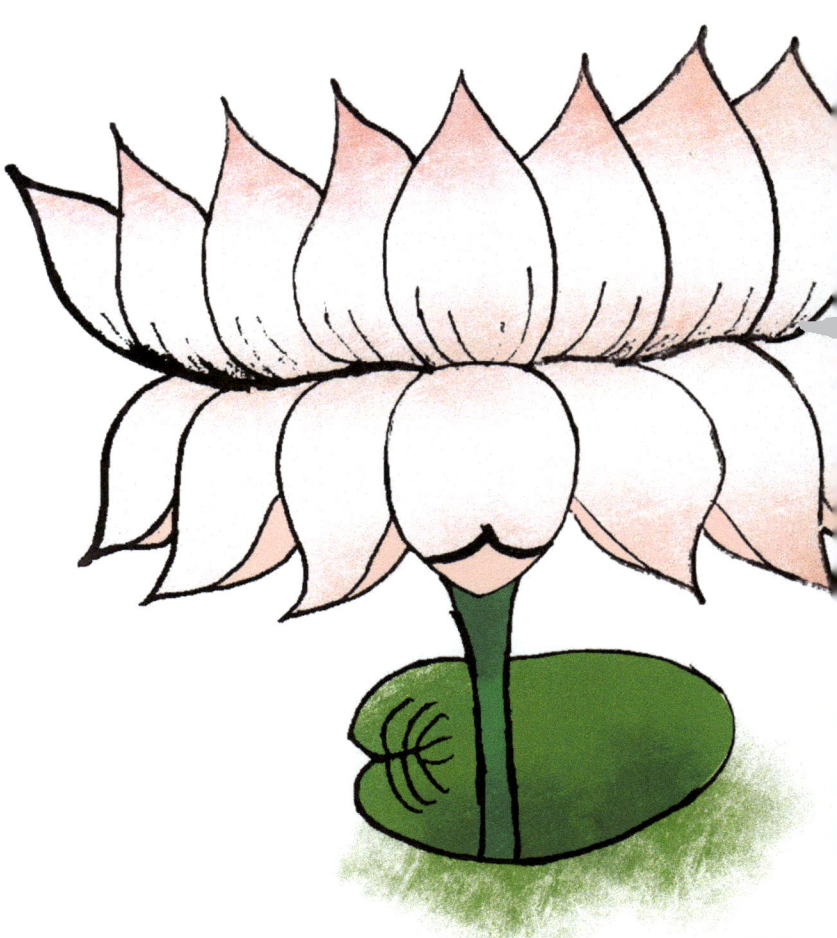

JUICY STUFF

Playing around
dancing
bright firelight of tejas
juicy and gorgeous ojas
the effervescent lifeforce
that is prana
together we bring everything alive
delving deep
into our new reality.

THE JUICY STUFF

Within everything we do, in our life experience and the bodymind, there is energy. Energy can be felt tangibly. Sometimes when we enter a room, it can feel awkward, heavy, light, strange or super comfortable. Energy is like love. We cannot see energy, but we can definitely experience it and know that it exists.

This is consciousness medicine. This is about bringing about change from within, not from external focus. We create our own change.

We have different energetic qualities that can be found in different ways within the bodymind. We saw this with the states of rajas and tamas (see page 47) and the doshas (see page 19). These different states are a direct result of our actions. Our actions are how we live, the food we eat, our activity levels, our mental focus, our environment, absolutely everything we experience and choose to do. This is the juicy stuff.

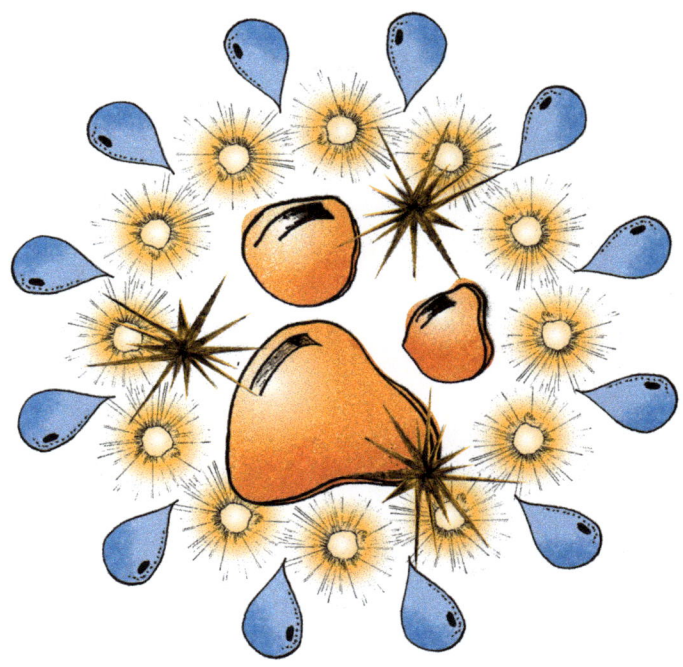

This is what drives us, what gives us that healthy glow, or not, if it's lacking. It's about living our life to its full potential and becoming the best version of ourselves, mentally, physically and emotionally. The best version of you that is possible in this lifetime, in this present moment. So what exactly is it and how can we have more of it? And what might affect it on a day-to-day basis? Can we have it all, health, wealth and happiness?

PRANA

Prana is often interpreted as life force. It is our vital essence. Prana arrives within us on the vehicle of the breath, in our environment and in our food. Every single body cell is said to contain prana. If you've ever been with someone and watched them take their last breath you have witnessed the leaving of prana from the physical form. As the last out-breath leaves the body so does the prana. There is a definitive moment of disconnect. Prana is associated with the vata dosha plus the air and ether elements.

TEJAS

Tejas is the inner spark. Is a twinkle in the eyes. An intelligence of spirit and intellect, your natural inherent intelligence. When our tejas is good we have a kind of inner, but also visible, bright and healthy glow. We are a bright spark. Tejas is associated with the pitta dosha plus the fire and water elements.

OJAS

Ojas is juicy. It is unctuous and supremely healthy, associated with our inner vitality, our physical and psychological resilience and our immunity to disease. When our ojas is good we feel grounded, supported, nurtured, can give to others and not deplete ourselves and we are holistically healthy, happy and free from disease. Ojas is associated with the kapha dosha plus the earth and water elements.

We keep the doshas and all these energetic qualities in balance by how we live our life. There is a lot of information in the previous chapters about specific practices to help with this. Below are some thoughts on these practices and the various aspects of our lives that may help these qualities evolve and thrive within us.

Mental focus

The mind is such an intangible yet also real entity for all of us. The mind is linked to our physical, and emotional states and can contribute to prevention or exacerbation of dis-ease in the physical body. How we learn to use or befriend the mind makes a vast difference to how we are in this world, as well as how we are in all regards of our existence in this lifetime. Practices such as meditation and mindfulness, yoga and focused breathing techniques all help us understand the mind better and therefore learn to live with it. Whatever thoughts come from the mind, we need to understand and know that we don't always need to respond or even listen to them. We can take some time out from our thoughts and thinking. If we can do this for a few minutes each day life can begin to feel a great deal more simple and peaceful.

Physical focus

The body was designed to move. I am not suggesting you run a marathon or scale a mountain. But do move your body every single day. If you find yourself at a desk or computer then get up at least once every hour and walk about, relax the shoulders, take some deep breaths. Notice any body parts that aren't feeling so great. Never ignore even the slightest sign of an

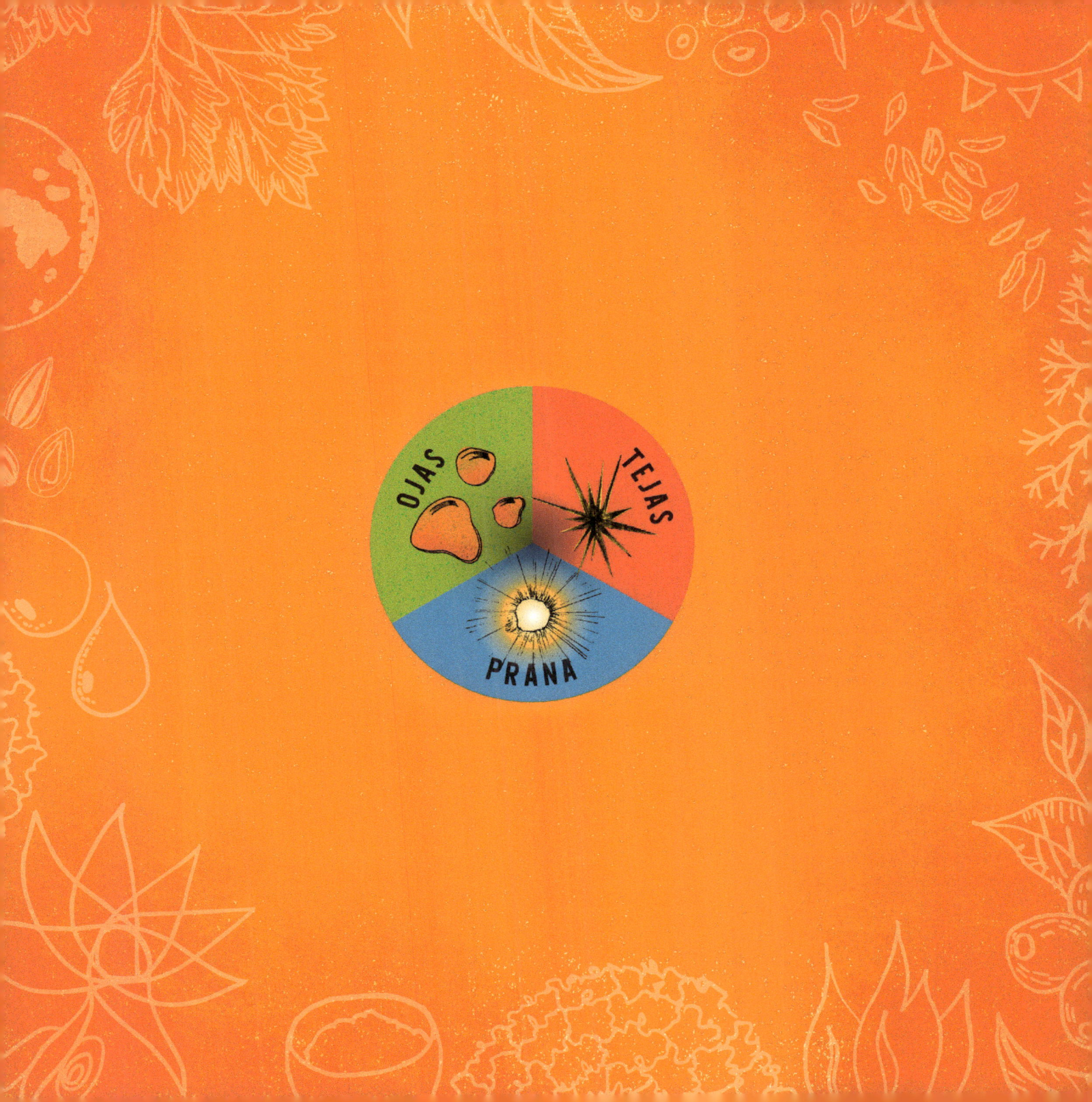

imbalance in the body. We seem to have developed a habit if something in the body is not quite right of calling this body part 'bad'. The body is not bad, it is trying to tell us things and we need to listen. So move the body daily, move it mindfully, slowly and notice how it is feeling. If you do notice that something isn't quite right then maybe investigate further, treat the body with kindness and do something about it, rather than leaving it to escalate.

Daily routine

I cannot emphasise enough the importance and positive impact of a good daily routine. When this was first suggested to me several years ago my initial reaction was... 'routine, blah, how boring'. I am now a total convert. I have discovered that I can travel and still maintain the routine and that this helps me stay healthy when travelling. I have also discovered that my sleep, energy levels, concentration and overall health are vastly improved and consistent as a result. I notice if I break the routine, for example by eating later, then I don't sleep so well and I feel sluggish the following day. Think about it. If a small child or even a puppy is fractious and agitated, what's the thing we instinctively tend to do? Put them into a good routine. We as adults are no different. When a client comes to me with a lot of health concerns I often see that insomnia is also an issue. Just by changing their daily routine they begin to sleep better. Because they are sleeping better their energy levels improve, their mind then begins to settle, they digest their food better. The benefits are many. It really never ceases to amaze me just how powerful this is. Do yourself a massive favour, if you do nothing else adapt the dinacharya, the daily routine (see page 22).

Food

After routine food is the most essential component here. In fact they are of equal importance. As I have already discussed food literally turns into, and becomes, the cells in our body. So we are completely made of what we eat. The energy in food is a massive consideration. I'm not against meat but do consider this: dead flesh versus vibrant green leaves. You can clearly see what will benefit the bodymind more and what contains the most prana, vibrant energy for the bodymind. Frozen and pre-packaged food is (obviously) not freshly prepared, so its energy will be less vibrant. In addition the way we prepare our food is of paramount importance. If we prepare food in a distracted way when in a bad mood it is unlikely to taste or look as good as when we are focused, full of love for the food and ourselves as well as whoever else we might be preparing it for. I, like perhaps many of you, often eat alone because I live alone. It's too easy to get lazy with food when you live alone I know. But please do take the same love and care over the food as you would if you were preparing a meal for dear friends.

You are your own best friend, so begin acting like it.

Remember, no one else can do this for you.

Environment

This can mean a myriad of things. Of course we want to care for the wider environment with our choice of detergents, food and packing choices, body products, travel and transport. So yes this is all a consideration. As well as this we want to be aware of our immediate everyday environment which we constantly inhabit. It's a kind of microcosm macrocosm approach, if we look after our immediate environment and everyone else begins to do the same then the wider environment will also begin to improve.

Consider your living space. As well as planet friendly, is it peaceful? Is it conducive to helping you to feel balanced? To enabling you to self-care? If you have a busy household with lots of people can you at least carve out a small corner and time for yourself each day? What about the location you live in, do you even like it there? Can you get access to nature, outdoors and greenery easily? If not can you introduce this somehow into your world? This is somewhat idyllic but humans thrive on fresh air, outdoors, nature, plus alone time for reflection. Notice how different you feel when you can access these things. If you don't do this regularly can you begin to plan to do this more? If this feels challenging focus on how this might feel when it happens, rather than any obstacles.

Other people and relationships

This is a big one! We can be (and are) totally responsible for ourselves, but what about other people? This may be people you are close to and live with, family members friends or work colleagues. We are constantly interacting with other people and having their energy thrown at us. Sometimes this can feel wonderful, at other times it might not be so great. One of my first ever yoga teachers, Jenni, said 'always water your own garden first'. Meaning that if we can learn to self-care as our priority, this helps our relationships with other people. We have more energy and clarity and are able to make better judgements in terms of our relationships as well as having more boundaries around what our own needs are. It is not selfish to do this, it's essential for our own health and well-being.

Connection

It's a disconnected world. You see so many people, heads down looking at screens, headphones in the ears, making no face-to-face or eye contact with other people. We seek connection on devices whilst missing potential for real human connection all around us every day. Say hello to strangers, smile at them and make eye contact, really see them as a person, just like you, trying to find their way in life as best they can. Let other cars out in traffic, smile as you do this. stop whilst driving to let people cross the road. Notice who is serving you in the shop, look them in the eye, smile, really see them and say thank you. Every now and then have a device free day, a digital detox. We are all just trying to find our way and we are all craving connection.

Our unique balance and character

We are all unique, we are all different from one another and yet, paradoxically, we are all working within these human limitations and in a similar structure of the bodymind. It is essential, if we are to travel through life relatively peacefully, to recognise that we all have different characters, different needs and priorities. A sense of understanding can arise just from that basic awareness of honouring one another's similarities and differences. In addition, we change as we journey through this life cycle. I am absolutely not the same character I was in my early twenties! And I am sure in ten years from now I will have evolved again. Don't be afraid to embrace this changing landscape for yourself and for others.

What is wealth?

Is wealth only financial? I am sure you are aware that it isn't. I am so fortunate to be abundant in good friends, natural beautiful landscape surrounding where I live, and more incredible beauty in the place where I stay in Kerala. I have a wealth of knowledge about wellness, how to prepare good food and how to keep myself healthy. This journey of wellness in turn gifts me so many different and creative life options. In addition, I have found the more I am able to let go of planning and plotting, the more abundance seems to arrive at my door. I am not financially wealthy, but I also never want for anything whatsoever. Allowing things to unfold creates this process of some kind of exchange with the universe. It is a trusting relationship with whatever you feel is going on, and it cannot be faked. Begin small, start to set gentle intentions and make lists. Also practice gratitude (see page 136), and notice what starts to slowly unfold.

Happiness and contentment

'Be grateful for whoever comes as each has been sent as a guide from beyond'. An insightful quote from 'The Guesthouse', a poem by Rumi.

Can we be content with whatever arises? We seem to have this inner drive to be eternally happy, gratified and fulfilled. This creates a sense of grasping and consuming. Because of the way we are programmed, particularly in the West, from an early age we look outside of ourselves to create the happiness we long for. Possessions, consumerism and distraction from reality are all endemic in our society today. Do these things make us truly happy? Surely true happiness is there even when you are not surrounded by all your stuff. If you lost everything right now, today, your home, all your belongings, your job, who would you then be? And could you be content and happy in another way, from deep inside? Can you be content and in awe at the sight of incredible luminous greens in spring, or at the cobalt blue of a summer sky, the taste of honey or the sound of a melody? What truly brings happiness? I am not suggesting you walk away from your life, but please do begin to notice the smaller things, the in-between moments, for this is where the real happiness truly lies. Herein lies true contentment, then, whatever comes, no one can take this away from you.

Let go of fear

In today's world there is a massive amount of fear, both individual and collective. Fear arises from confusion, information from the media, government agendas, being stuck in a place where you don't feel you can be truly yourself and feeling trapped. When we live in fear we are constantly in a state of flight and flight, the bodymind is full of tension and this exacerbates the risk of dis-ease. Fear affects every single body system, our sense of perception and our cognition. It is not easy to let go of this fearful state and no-one can do this for you. Letting go of fear can feel risky and unfamiliar. When in fear we do not make rational decisions, because we are in pure survival mode. We prefer to stay with the familiar and the comfortable, to go with majority and not be in the minority, which is what feels safe. This means that nothing can change. Letting go of fear takes time, it's kind of like learning to swim. You can dip your toe into the water here and there, maybe even paddle up to your knees, start to doggy paddle perhaps, but at some point you just have to get in, or maybe you will be pushed. Then you really learn to swim. When you begin to focus on what is actually real, on nature, rhythms and cycles, energy and emotion, then you will begin to let go of all that is not real. The more you focus the more real things become and the fear melts away. You realise that everything was ok all along. There is no need to feel afraid. Beyond fear you will find freedom.

Face

Everything

And

Rise

Opportunity from serendipity

When we let go of fear we can allow things to unfold. Keep things simple. This simplicity can feel complex for us at first because it is so unfamiliar. Can you focus just on what you are doing and nothing else? Stop multitasking, and do just one thing at a time, do it well and only once completed move onto the next thing. Begin to notice seemingly irrelevant or random coincidences. These are opportunities. People often say to me that I am very lucky. When I could say that I have suffered massive misfortune having lost my partner, home and business several years ago. So how can I be lucky? Because I see the opportunity in the serendipity. I notice when things come along, and I try them out. Not everything is something I want or need to hold onto long term, but some things are. By creating a simpler less complex life, we have more time to notice what is going on, and to create opportunity from the serendipity.

SERENDIPITY IS THE EXPERIENCE OF FINDING SOMETHING JOYFUL IN THAT WHICH CAME UNEXPECTEDLY.

Life isn't always a bed of roses

Life is sometimes tough, really extraordinarily tough. Things we could never have imagined happen to us and to our loved ones and life changes forever in the blink of an eye. All the more reason to make the best job we can of being here. The Buddha talks about acceptance (of suffering) and non-grasping. These are very difficult concepts in our reality. We will suffer, this is an inevitable element of life. We do not want to suffer because it is beyond uncomfortable, and we shy away from this discomfort. We use things, possessions, foods, behaviours, substances to distract us from our suffering. This strategy does not work, it does not make the suffering go away. So we do these things more and more until we literally can't hear or feel or experience ourselves thinking or being. And yet the suffering remains. What can we do? We can learn to make friends with the suffering. You may wonder why on earth you would want to do this. The suffering is a part of you, it is a part of all of us. The sooner you get used to this idea the better. How do we befriend the suffering? By stripping away all the layers slowly and with love to reveal what lies beneath. The practices and techniques described in this book are a beginning. When we eventually get though all the layers of illusion and perception, we find beneath it all that we were ok all along. Beneath all this crazy mixed up madness we are actually a peaceful and content being, a sattvic soul.

Effortless effort

It may feel like it is a big effort to achieve this state of what we call sattva. The answer is well, yes and no. It is in no way straightforward, and yet it is also the most straightforward thing we ever need to do. The concept is one of effortless effort. If we strive to reach this goal of peace and equanimity then the very action of striving will also stop us from reaching it, because you see we are doing the very thing we need to stop. So put into place the routine, the sattvic food, the cleansing, self-care, meditation, simplicity, let go of fear and embrace serendipity. We need to allow it to unfold, rather than try to make it happen. And it does. This requires patience. These approaches are not a quick fix. We allow the layers to begin ever so tenderly to peel themselves away. We begin to know our true self and to feel, see and experience what is actually real. This can be a challenge, quite often for people around you more than for you as they feel you may be going 'weird' or changing. This process can feel like a sacrifice of regular everyday life and everything we have ever known. Only you can take this journey and decide if it is for you and once you are on your way, you will discover that lots of us are there right beside you.

Practices that can help to cultivate prana, tejas and ojas

As well as the food we eat, cleansing and having a good daily routine and other practices can help us increase, nurture and hold onto these energetic life-enhancing qualities.

Yoga

In the West yoga has been largely commercialised and mainstreamed to appeal to a wide consumer market. It has become a massive industry. This has, to some extent resulted in some people feeling they can't 'do' yoga, or it isn't for them, because they don't fit the stereotype on the magazine cover. Let's get something straight here: yoga is not about whether you can fling your leg over your shoulder, it is about peace of mind though the vehicle of the body. Yoga can be adapted to suit absolutely everyone without exception.

The physical practice of yoga, from my perspective, also embraces the philosophical aspects.

A physical practice embraces ahimsa (non-harming) to oneself, physically as well as psychologically. It should have a principle of satya (truth), being honest with oneself about what we need from the practice - this isn't always what we want! Consider what your practice is about today. Can you meet these needs in a non-judgmental way and thus also bring into the practice an attitude of aparigraha (non-grasping).

Practice should be done in an intelligent and logical way that is suitable for your body as it is today, with or without the guidance of a teacher. This practice is about honouring yourself, body, mind, emotions, spirit and energy, with your yoga. We use the physical to delve into the psychological. Fully focusing on the breath within the asana (posture and movement) practice in order to bring about a feeling of santosha (contentment), an acceptance of the bodymind as it is, here, right now in the moment. Then to have an attitude of ishvara pranidhana (devotion), towards oneself, towards this ancient practice and the lineage, to all the ancient texts, and the rishis and sages from which it all came.

It is important that you find a yoga teacher who you resonate with, that you feel understands you and the practice they offer you. If you haven't found that person yet, keep looking. They are out there somewhere.

Please don't undervalue or underestimate yoga. It is such a precious, beautiful gift to yourself and to mankind. Practice pranayama (breathing exercises) after the asana (postures and movement), always. Calm the mind. Create for the bodymind a place of peace, of complete equanimity, sattva, balance. Breathe, focus, concentrate, and then sit still, allow yourself to just be for a while.

The mind is like a monkey that has been stung by a scorpion, looking for a black cat in a dark room, that isn't there.

**NOWHERE TO BE,
NOTHING TO DO,
JUST BREATHE.**

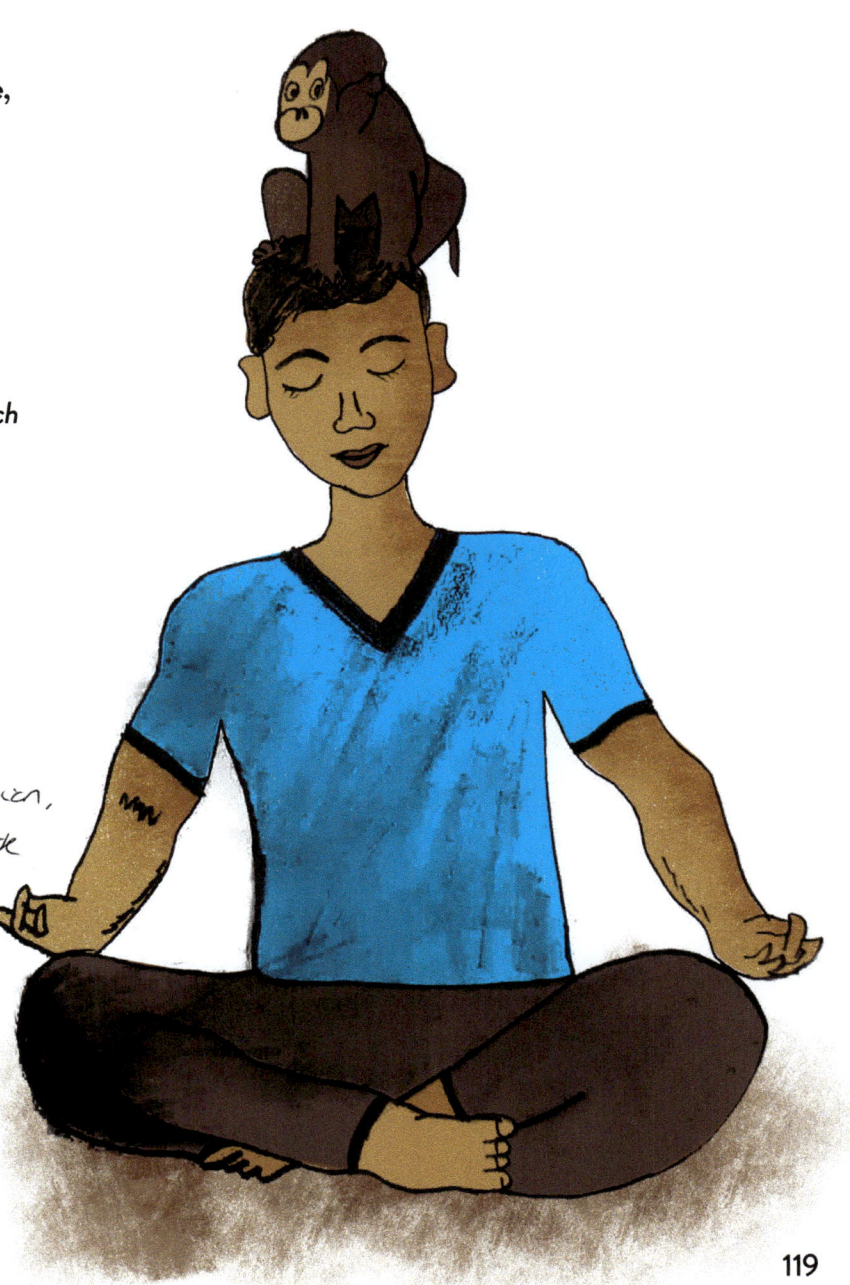

Meditation

People often say they are unable to meditate. When asked they will generally say this is because their mind is too busy. Newsflash! Everyone's mind is busy. The art of sitting and noticing helps us begin to understand this, and we need to begin to accept it. So please have no expectations. Meditation also takes practice. You are unlikely to become enlightened in five minutes time out in the midst of a busy life. We can do our best by following the practices I have talked about and by using a simple technique for maybe five minutes each day, more if possible. Ideally this is done first thing in the morning. Partly because we are less likely to get our attention diverted then and also because stuff happens during the day and distracts us and we don't then get around to it. Follow the steps below and see what happens.

YOUR ARE BEGINNING TO KNOW YOURSELF, BEYOND THE BODYMIND.
YOU ARE BEGINNING TO KNOW THE SATTVIC SOUL.

A simple meditation

Sit comfortably. It is not advisable to lie down as you may fall asleep.

Ensure you feel supported, you can sit in a chair, on the floor, on a cushion, whatever works for you. Use cushions, blankets anything you need.

Have some water to hand in case you need it.

You need to feel alert yet relaxed.

Check your forehead, jaw and shoulders are relaxed.

Now observe what happens next.

Notice what arises. Watch the thoughts.

Sit with whatever comes and patiently observe. Keep watching.

Do not strive to change or fix anything.

Know that it will pass, even if it feels difficult or pleasant, everything is constantly changing. So don't try to change anything, just observe.

Practice aparigraha (non-grasping) and see what arises, with a gentle kindness. Allow it all to ebb and flow.

See if you can be aware of feeling rather than thoughts and thinking.

Feeling not thinking.

Find within this practice an acceptance, a sukkah (sweet spot), a place of gratitude, of svadyaya (continual learning), a journey into the self, through the vehicle of the body and breath and beyond the mind.

Practice, observe and then let it all be.

INGREDIENTS, EQUIPMENT AND COOKING NOTES

Food is an integral part of this whole process. There are some ingredients and kitchen equipment that will definitely enhance your whole cookery experience. Some things can be expensive, but I have also offered more economical alternatives as not everyone is able to spend a huge amount and it's actually not necessary to do so. It is also always worth checking what is around secondhand, especially with blenders and the more pricey stuff.

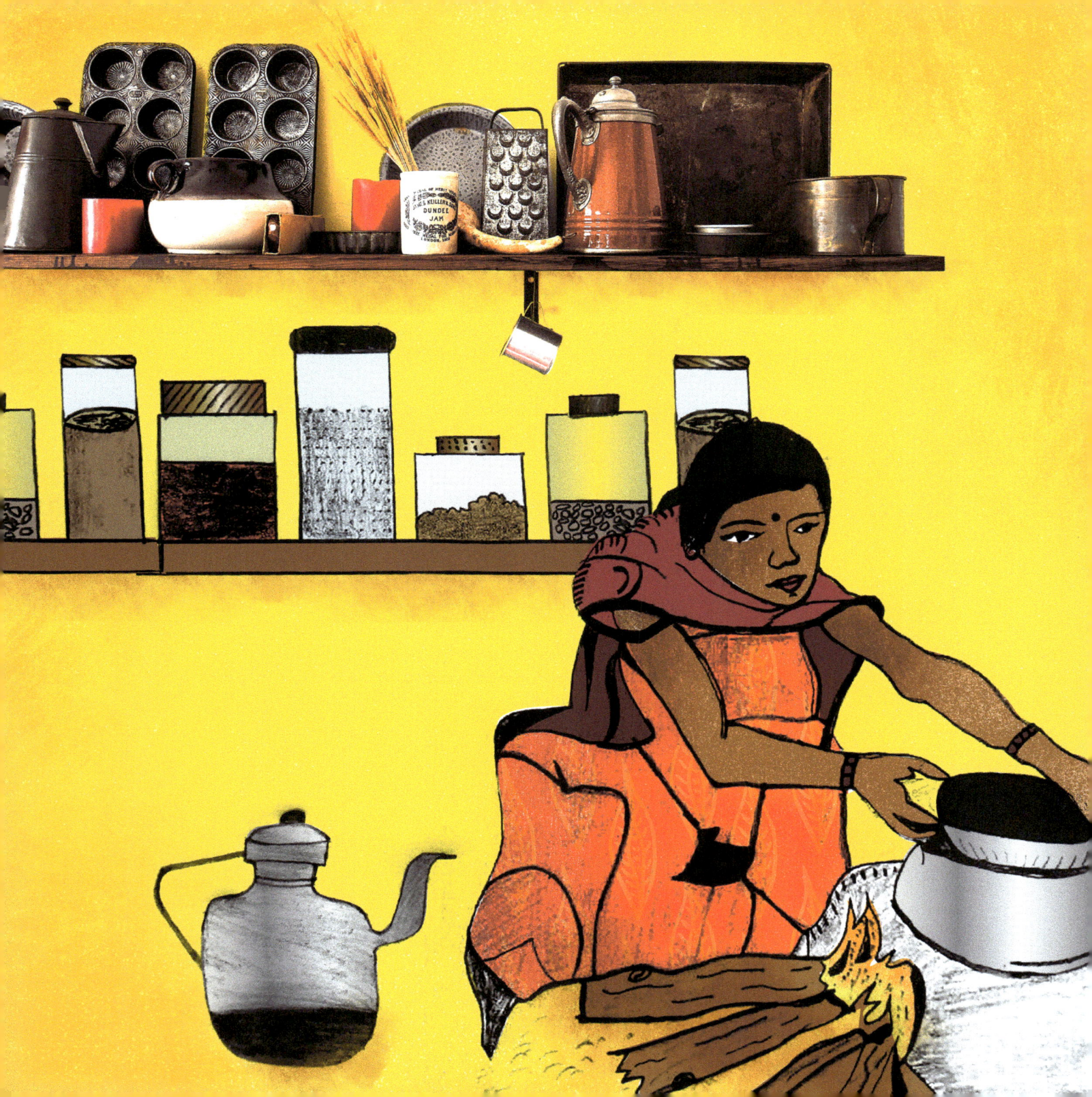

ESSENTIAL EQUIPMENT

The cooker: As long as you have some kind of hob you can create lots of lovely dishes. At one stage I lived somewhere with a very shared space and completely without any kind of kitchen. I cooked everything on a two-ring plug in hob and it worked really well. You absolutely do not need a big fancy kitchen and cooker. I never use a microwave and only occasionally use an oven, probably because I still don't have a full-size oven, but this keeps me super creative!

One really good chopping knife: Keep it sharp! Worth spending as much as you are able to on this as you will use it a lot.

One smaller knife: I use an outdoor gardening knife as hardly ever use this one so just grab something multipurpose.

Good size sturdy chopping board: Doesn't need to be expensive, just needs to do the job and have space for everything you are chopping.

Stick blender: For soups and so on. You can get these quite cheaply. If possible one that also has a small container attachment.

Jug blender: When I was completely skint I found a super cheap alternative for around £30 and it totally did the job. If you're feeling flush you can look at more expensive options.

Wok: Or stir fry pan, with a lid is nice but not essential.

Saucepan with lid: For cooking rice and grains.

Small pan: For milk

Grater: For veg and also for ginger, so with different sized holes.

Wooden spoons: And implements, rather than plastic or metal.

Sieve and colander: Self-explanatory.

NICE BUT UNESSENTIAL EQUIPMENT

Pestle and mortar: A good big heavy one that you can really get grinding in!

Food processor: The ultimate time saver if wanting to do loads of grating or mixing, but definitely not essential.

Nice teapot: With a filter for herb teas. Bit of a luxury!

Measuring jug and scales: You can use cups etc to roughly measure instead. You can get fancy cup measures, but really any regular cup is ok as long as you are consistent and use the same cup throughout a recipe so it all adds up.

Pressure cooker: Really super helpful with soups and dried pulses. A bit scary at first. When you get used to the way it works it may become an essential.

Water filter: This is kind of essential but not a total priority if not affordable so I've put it here. However please be aware of and research the benefits of filtering your water and consider this when you can. Once you have it only use filtered water for drinking and cooking.

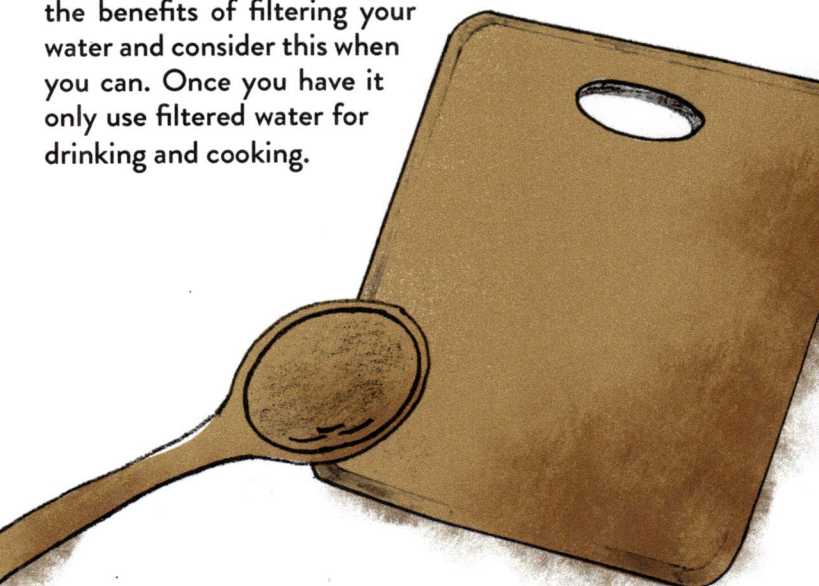

FAVOURITE FOODS

Lots of dried stuff here so in an emergency, even without fresh vegetables, you can create something tasty and nutritious. This includes dried pulses which require soaking and then cooking, this can take ages if you don't have a pressure cooker. These days I try to source organic and sustainable ingredients if possible. In the past I have managed to get by with whatever I could afford at the time. These dried foods are super nutritious, filling and so cheap, as well as long lasting in the store cupboard. You don't need to buy all this at once, just as you need for each recipe and slowly build it up as you go.

Pulses, beans, dried, soaked and pressure cooked or tinned? I prefer to pre-cook all dried beans by soaking and then pressure cooking. You can of course use tinned pulses if you prefer and they are handy if you need to be speedy. But be aware that the nutritional benefits are not as great and the taste of dried when prepared is much more wholesome somehow.

Black bean juice: The benefits of black beans are multiple. Try getting dried beans and soaking them overnight before pressure cooking them to use in a recipe. They are much more delicious this way. In addition, when cooking dried black beans, you end up with an unctuous thick black broth that is incredibly beneficial when drank on its own.

Chopping vegetables. Vegetables are full of vital energy (prana). When we hack away at them without thoughtful awareness we deplete this energy. When we ingest them in this state we deprive ourselves of the full beneficial effects of the food. Do, for example, take a carrot, wash it lovingly and pat it dry. Ask yourself, do I really need to peel this? Then instead of chopping straight across slice it at an angle, as you would if you were sharpening a pencil with a knife, continue this for the whole length of the carrot. Consider the direction in which the carrot grows to move towards the light of the sun and see if you can respect this in your preparation.

Try and use this approach with all vegetables, it's trickier with some but always possible. It may feel time consuming at first but you'll soon adjust and it becomes quire natural and incredibly satisfying. Plus the food somehow tastes better.

Nuts and seeds, soaking and toasting. Seeds are seeds, nuts are also seeds - think about it! They fall to the ground from the plant if left unharvested, and they grow. They are powerhouses of nutritional energy and 'good fat'. When a seed is raw it is in the perfect state to sprout and grow. When it is ingested in this state (as it would be by say a bird) it is therefore not easy to properly digest (think about sweetcorn for example). Therefore it is recommended that all nuts and seeds are either soaked in water, preferably overnight but if you're in a rush or forget just pour boiling water over and leave for at least one hour. Alternatively they can be toasted. Nuts are easier toasted in a warm oven, around 150°C for ten minutes, keep an eye on them as they have a habit of burning as soon as you turn your back! Seeds are scrumptious toasted in a dry frying pan. Great served with savoury dishes, porridge, all sorts of things, or as a stand alone snack. Incidentally the gold standard is to soak and then toast seeds if you have the time and the inclination!

Toasted seeds

1. Warm the pan then add the seeds, if using several different types toast them separately.

2. Keep gently and patiently moving them around and they will slight brown on the edges and smell amazing.

3. Serve immediately or leave to cool and store in a glass jar until required.

A note about storage. Try not to store food in plastic containers or packets. If you can use glass jars, save them once you're finished with whatever is inside and reuse. Rice can be bought in bulk in paper sacks if you have space. Spices prefer to be kept in a shady or darker space. You can line it all up on shelves and it looks beautiful as well as being accessible and easy to grab and use.

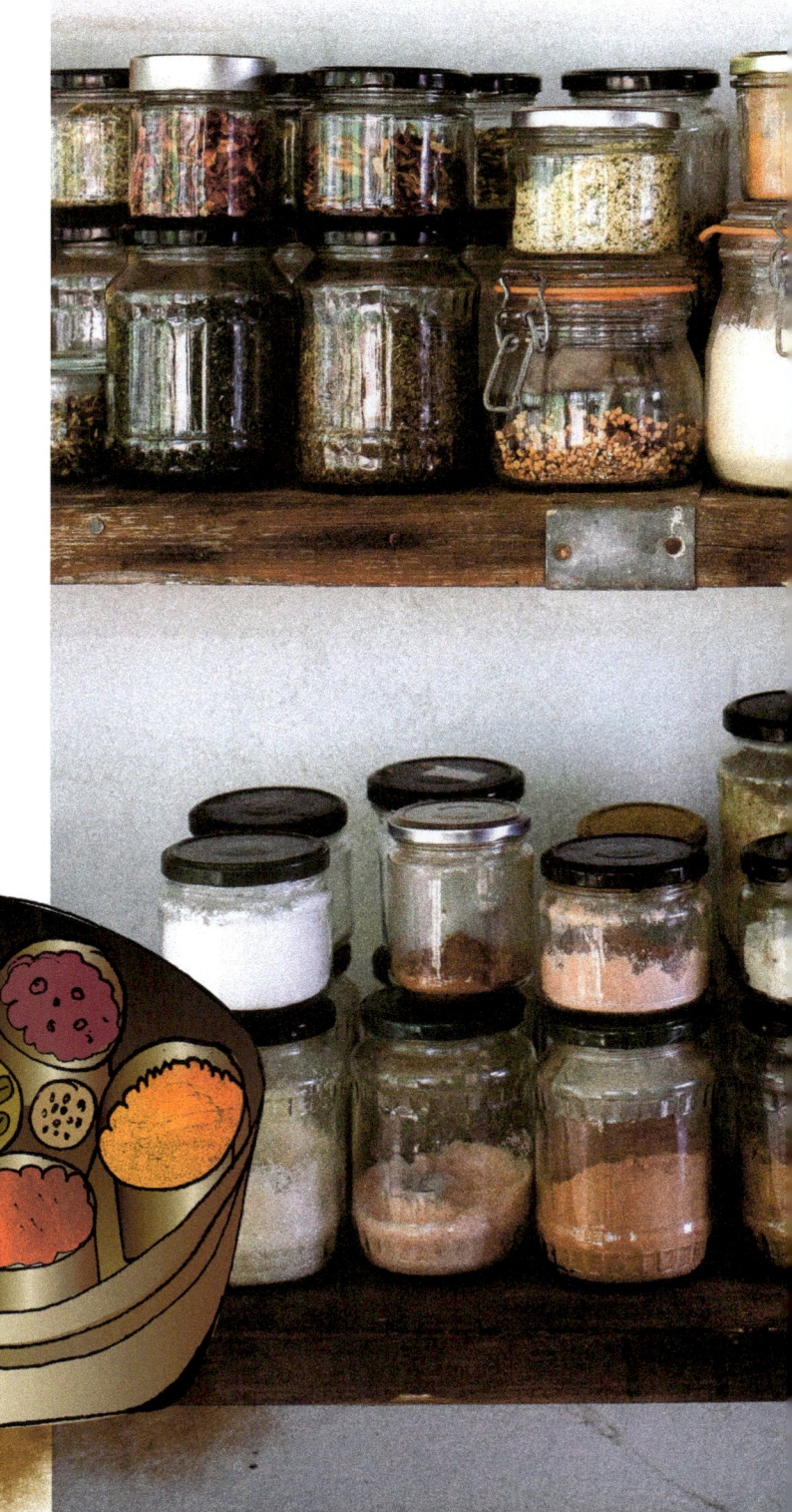

STORE CUPBOARD	GRAINS	PULSES	NUTS/SEEDS
ESSENTIALS	Rice, short grain and long grain brown as well as white basmati Oats for porridge	Mung (sometimes spelt Moong) daal is the ultimate essential, small yellow lentils (not split yellow peas)	Seeds: sunflower, sesame, pumpkin
GOOD BASIC	Quinoa, various colours, all are good	Lentils: red, green and other lentils of choice. Be aware that the red and mung (above) go mushy and others do not, so they have different uses.	Nuts: walnuts, cashew nuts, almonds
ONLY AS REQUIRED	Amaranth, bulgar wheat, cous cous, pasta	Chickpeas, black beans, aduki beans, black eyes beans. Nice to keep a small variety.	As you wish: hempseed, flaxseed, poppy seed, linseed, pistachios, brazils

SPICES	OTHER THINGS
Cumin (seed and ground), coriander (seed and ground), fennel, asafoetida (hing), turmeric, cardamom (seed and ground), ginger (fresh root if possible), black mustard seeds, black onion seed, cinnamon, nutmeg, curry leaves, black pepper, salt	Fats: Ghee, olive oil, sesame oil, coconut oil. Optionally, hemp oil, black cumin oil. Local honey Alternative sweeteners: rice syrup, date syrup, maple syrup
As you wish (and depending on your constitution), chilli, fenugreek, garlic, caraway	Soya type sauce, tamari is delicious and is also gluten free Mustard Balsamic and other vinegars for dressings Tahini (sesame seed paste)
Dried herbs as you wish (fresh are generally better if possible)	Fermented foods, you may wish to explore this more, kimchi, sauerkraut, kombucha, kefir, curd (yoghurt)

FRESH AND SIMPLE

Throw away things you haven't used that are looking a bit faded and jaded.

Notice what you tend to use more of and source this in bulk.

Store things in a beautiful way that makes things easy to find, open shelves are great for this as you can see everything without rummaging about.

If you live alone or even if there are just two of you don't buy too many vegetables at once as they then sit and go mushy when not used. They can get wasted. Buy vegetables as you need and plan to use them.

Buy what is in season. Learn about seasonal foods local to you. There is usually a large amount of seasonal produce so it is cheaper, healthier, tastes much better and has many more nutritional benefits.

fresh, seasonal, local.

SATTVIC SOUL

Love yourself
I give you the skill
you must practice
trust your perception
you must trust yourself
to do this you must love yourself
do you love yourself?

IT'S ALL ABOUT LOVE

If we are caring for someone we love then we want the best for them, we desire them to be happy, healthy and whole in their experience and enjoyment of life. We make sure, as much as we can, they have the best of everything. We wish for them to live a long, happy and peaceful life.

Do we ever stop for long enough to wish this or to practice this for ourselves? Do we love ourselves, and how easy is this? The recipes and rituals described here are all acts of self-love and self-care. These are practical things that you can do everyday. In a society where being focused on ourselves, on our own physical and emotional needs, can be labelled as selfish or self-obsessed, this is not always an easy path to choose to take. We are stepping away from ordinary everyday life and ways of being. Sometimes this way of viewing health is called 'alternative' and yet this is an ancient art, the original healthcare system, an imbedded wisdom that has been around for literally thousands of years. So it is not so unfamiliar, and when we embrace it there is a real sense of comfort, of inner knowing. In the welcoming back of these rhythms and cycles we connect on a deeper level with ourselves. Beyond the distractions of regular life, beyond artificial agendas and ego driven expectations. We dive deep into our past, we walk alongside our ancestors, into nature, into the wilderness, into the ancient ways. We begin to feel better somehow. We begin to feel more at home, at peace and a sense of true belonging. This is real. This is not the false superficial belonging that we all crave and seek on a daily basis. This is authentic and true and beautiful, and it is all yours if you choose it. If you can begin to love yourself.

The word sattvic literally means essence. It represents mental strength, a calm peaceful energy, balance and equanimity in the bodymind. The sattvic soul state comes from these practices, from this way of being and from loving ourselves. When in this sattvic state we can view a clear version of reality much more naturally, without all the layers in the way. Sattva is said to represent truth, knowledge and wisdom in its greatest sense.

To come into this state of sattva we explore all the layers of our being, embrace all the cycles of nature and align ourselves unreservedly.

We need to be focused and strong. We constantly choose our mental, physical and emotional reactions which determine our state of mind. We have a choice about how we respond to every situation, every event, every circumstance. We create expectations for ourselves and then suffer as a result of our responses. We need to let these expectations go. Our deep consciousness, our sattvic soul, remains untouched by it all, we must learn to care for, nourish, nurture and connect with it. It is forever peaceful. This connection gives us strength and power. In this state we take control of the bodymind. We become sattvic.

We can see in this final diagram how everything is interrelated. We can understand how if one element or part of our routine becomes unsynchronised from its cycle it will create an imbalance throughout our whole being.

As we move from youth into adulthood if we retain too much kapha (earth and water) in the bodymind we will feel sluggish, unmotivated, have excess mucus and maybe even suffer from depression. On the other hand the vata (air and ether) in excess at the inappropriate life-stage can create anxiety, insomnia and ungroundedness. In its place, later in life, the vata gifts us with increased insight and wisdom. Earlier in life if fully in balance, kapha helps us to feel grounded and secure whilst growing and learning. Everything has its place in this system. These elements are meant to exist in a rhythm. They're also affected by the climate, so we may notice we feel the cold more and need to rebalance ourselves at certain times of year or even at particular phases of the moon or times of day. If the elements shift so do our energies of prana tejas and ojas, this can then create an imbalance in the bodymind which leads to dis-ease. We might be more of a morning or evening person. We are all unique, and yet we all have in common these naturally arising ways of being, the innate capacity to tune into nature and to ourselves.

This is a beautiful science. It comes from the earth. We are made of the earth. Our DNA is not so dissimilar to that of plants. This is largely why it works. These are simple practices. They are over 5000 years old. This way of being is a truly magical and ancient art.

Balanced
Feeling easeful
Open to receive
whatever comes.
Filled with gratitude
Bodymind and soul
Perfect equanimity
Grounded yet spacious
Peaceful
Accepting whatever is
as it is meant to be.
Undisturbed
Deeply joyful.
So very calm
Yet fully awake.
Extraordinarily aware,
an inner knowing.
Beyond the ordinary everyday
Gently transcending
Connected.
Sattvic Soul

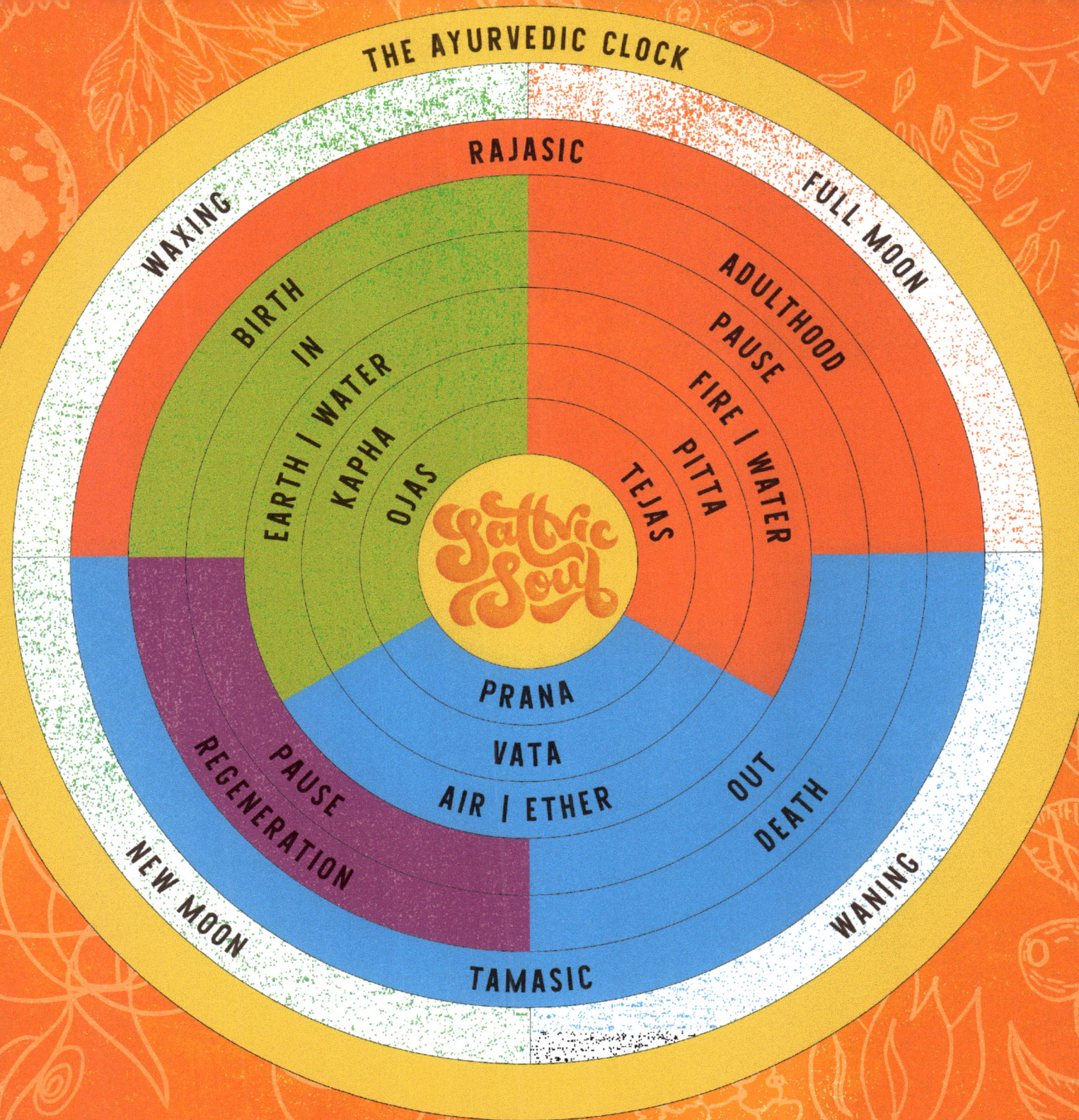

GLOSSARY OF WORDS

Below is an alphabetical list of words used throughout the book that may have been unfamiliar to you. Please use this to keep looking things up as you need.

Ahimsa ~ Non-harming.

Aparigraha ~ Non-grasping.

Asafoetida ~ Also called hing. This is a dried powdered root used in ayurvedic cookery that gives a pungency to replace the taste of onions. It is also helpful for digestion.

Asana ~ Yoga postures, the literal translation is 'steady comfortable seat'.

Ashwahandga ~ An ayurvedic herb that is rejuvenative.

Ayurveda ~ Ayur=life Veda=science. A complete system for maintaining wellness in body and mind.

Ama ~ Toxins in the body. Caused by unsuitable food, lack of movement, lifestyle and routine, environmental factors and our psychological and emotional states.

Bodymind ~ A concept that the body and mind are the same thing.

Dharma ~ This can be translated as, right direction or rightful duty. Your dharma means your purpose in life. Your dharma is your true calling, what you were put here to do.

Dinacharya ~ The cyclical daily routine according to ayurvedic principles.

Dosha ~ A specific constitutional state in the practice of ayurveda. There are three dosha types, kapha, pitta and vata and we are all a combination of all three in varying amounts.

Dukkha ~ Suffering.

Guna ~ Three different types of energetic state. Rajas, high energy. Tamas, low energy. Sattvic, balanced.

Ishvara pranidhana ~ Devotion in terms of a focus for spiritual practice.

Kapalbhati ~ A breathing technique that is rapid, heating and cleansing, also thought to move energy around the body. Caution in cases of high blood pressure and vertigo, plus pregnancy and any abdominal disturbance or menstrual bleeding. Good to learn with a qualified teacher.

Kapha dosha ~ Combined of earth and water. Qualities of heavy, grounded, lubricating. Seen as loving, stable, grasping.

Kosha ~ Layer or sheath. There are five koshas or layers to the human form. Anamaya (food or physical body), pranamaya (energy or breath body), manamaya (thinking mind), vijnanamaya (intuition and imagination) and anandamaya (bliss).

Maca ~ A powdered root from South America, with rejuvenative hormone balancing qualities.

Moringa ~ An ayurvedic herb that has many benefits including being nutrient dense and highly bioavailable.

Namaste ~ A gesture of greeting one another, not a superficial gesture but a way of showing respect and that you are equal to one another. It is used with all people one meets, from young and old to friends and strangers.

Nasaya oil ~ An oil specifically for use in the nose after cleansing practices. Great for respiratory health and infection prevention, as per neti (below).

Neti ~ The practice of washing out the nostrils with warm salt water. Extremely beneficial for respiratory and sinus health, hay fever prevention, allergy sufferers and general prevention of respiratory infections.

Ojas ~ Energy that is nurturing and nourishing, giving good immunity and a general good state of health.

Pitta dosha ~ Combined of fire and water. Qualities are hot, intense, transformative. Seen as creating change, focused, hot-headed.

Prakruti ~ Your constitutional balance at conception and you 'blueprint' for life. Determined by your parents, the time of conception, place of conception, climate and environmental factors.

Prana ~ Vital life force, life energy. Very linked with the breath but also present in all living things.

Pranayama ~ Breathing practices that move and alter the prana (above).

Santosha ~ Contentment.

Sattvic ~ To be in balance, to be healthy, happy, feeling at peace with and sense of harmony and well-being. This can apply to food, to ourselves in our body and mind or to our environment.

Satya ~ Truth.

Soul ~ Somehow we are aware that within us there is an inner wisdom, and sense of knowing, an essence that reaches beyond the everyday. This may be called the soul. The soul is always sattvic (above).

Sukkha ~ Sweet spot, happiness, an excellent space.

Svadyaya ~ Continual learning.

Tejas ~ Energy that gives a kind of inner spark and intelligence.

Triphala ~ An ayurvedic herbal mixture containing three fruits, haritaki, bibhitaki and amalaki. Regulates and supports digestion and body systems.

Vata dosha ~ Combined of air and ether. Qualities are cold, dry, light. Seen as movement, imagination, creativity, constantly changeable.

Vrikruti ~ Your constitutional state as you are right now, today. Influenced by food, environment, climate and life experience.

Yoga ~ Often seen as a physical posture practice, traditional yoga also includes breathing and meditation practices. Yoga is often translated as meaning 'union.' This can be viewed as union of breath and body or union with a higher power.

Yoga Nidra ~ A form of deep methodical relaxation. A practice that produces feelings of deep inner calm and relaxation, helps to calm the mind and alleviate feelings of restlessness and anxiety.

RECIPES AND RITUALS INDEX

Below is an index of recipes and rituals found in this book.

In a way a recipe is a kind of ritual - the consideration of what to eat, of how to nurture ourselves with food, of preparing food mindfully and lovingly. This approach to life is very ritualistic in its routines and recommendations. This gives us a sense of stability and comfort, whatever may be happening. We can return to these simple beautiful offerings time after time and they will always be here for us.

Aduki beetroot stew - **page 64**

Almond coconut prasad - **page 83**

Apple, stewed - **page 54**

Aromatic sweet potato and tofu - **page 64**

Baked beans - **page 63**

Banana bread - **page 82**

Bean chilli - **page 63**

Beetroot cashew dip - **page 76**

Beetroot rose latte - **page 87**

Beetroot raita - **page 78**

Beetroot Sauté - **page 70**

Beetroot soup - **page 79**

Blessing food - **page 100**

Bombay mix salad - **page 60**

Buckwheat pancakes - **page 55**

Cashew cream - **page 85**

Cassoulet, vegan ayurvedic - **page 66**

Chai style tea - **page 88**

Chocolate almond dates - **page 83**

Chocolate torte - **page 85**

Churna spice mix for each dosha - **page 33**

Churna spice mix porridge - **page 54**

Cleansing - **page 99**

Coconut curry sauce - **page 67**

Courgette dip - **page 78**

Digestive tea - **page 86**

Dressing, classic - **page 75**

Dressing, tahini and lemon - **page 75**

Dressing, oily mustard - **page 75**

Dressing, turmeric - **page 76**

Dukkah (nutty healthy snack) - **page 73**

Fire Cider - **page 105**

Full moon ritual - **page 42**

Ginger turmeric pickle - **page 73**

Ginger turmeric tea - **page 86**

Golden milk - **page 86**

Gomassio (sesame salt) - **page 71**

Green tea salad - **page 58**

Healing broth - **page 105**

Hearty soup - **page 80**

Hemp seed mayo - **page 75**

Humous - **page 77**

Indian roast chickpeas - **page 70**

Kale and broccoli with satay - page 60

Kitchari - page 102

Lassi - page 88

Lemon courgettes - page 62

Masala omelette - page 55

Meal in a bowl, soup and extras - page 80

Meditation, simple - page 120

Meditation, gratitude - page 136

Moon bath, full moon - page 43

Moon bath, new moon - page 45

Muffins (Stephen's) - page 83

New moon cleanse - page 108

New moon ritual - page 44

Oat cookies - page 82

Poached pears - page 57

Porridge - page 54

Potatoes - page 62

Potatoes and greens - page 68

Rejuvenating tonic - page 104

Rice, sweet - page 106

Roast root veg - page 70

Roasted stone fruit - page 57

Slaw - page 78

Sleep tea - page 87

Smoothie, ojas - page 89

Smoothie, green energising - page 89

Smoothie, decadent and definitely not ayurvedic - page 89

Stir fried greens - page 68

Sweet potato soup - page 79

Tahini cream - page 78

Tamari seeds - page 74

Tibetan raita - page 77

Tofu and kale with tahini dressing - page 61

Ume radishes - page 71

Vegetable rice - page 67

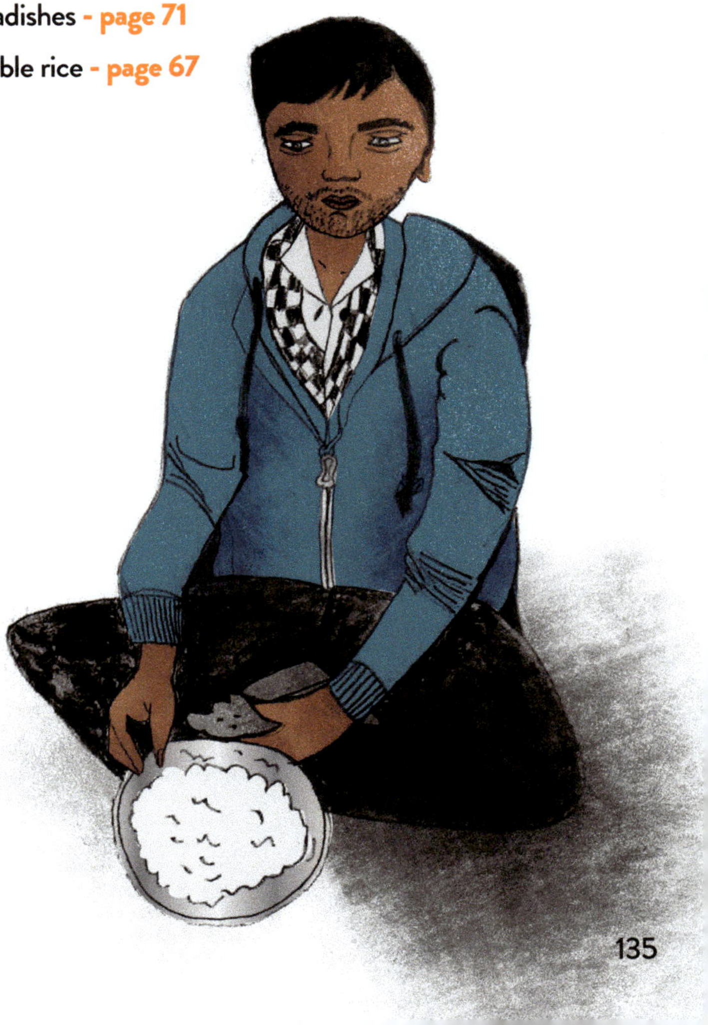

GRATITUDE

A beautiful meditation is the practice of gratitude. I learned this particular practice for the very first time in Kathmandu. In addition to the practice described below I would like to acknowledge and offer gratitude to some very special people, without whom this creation and collection of thoughts would not have been possible.

Sophie Maliphant, the incredible designer and illustrator of this book, responsible for helping to bring to life Sattvic Soul and not least being a wonderful friend and an incredibly accurate interpreter of the dreams and imaginings in my mind.

Jenna Richards, such a patient editor and grammar checker as well as an incredible friend who I met some years ago through yoga.

Ashma Dahal, in Kathmandu, co-illustrator with Sophie, interpreting my dreams from a magical place which is very close to my heart.

Stephen Brandon, who is my primary teacher in ayurveda and yoga. His depth and breadth of knowledge constantly and consistently guides me, as does his belief in me, which enables me to fully embody these practices with complete authenticity.

Sunita Passi, whose vibrancy and creativity with ayurveda is forever inspirational. A true visionary and a very wonderful friend.

Shibu Krishna, who found me when I was lost and showed me the way. A very dear friend in Kerala, practicing ayurveda in the place where it all began.

Terry Crockett, my late partner and best friend. He always believed in me wholeheartedly. Although physically gone he continues to guide and inspire me.

The Sangha, all of my amazing and supportive friends and clients who continuously tolerate my total unwavering obsession with ayurveda. There are too many to mention. I am so very thankful for each and every one of you.

GRATITUDE MEDITATION PRACTICE

The focus of this gratitude practice can be anything at all. For the purposes of this particular offering I am using rice - when I did it in Kathmandu it was about the clothes we were wearing.

I have a bit of a thing about rice. It is eaten all over the world and sold very cheaply in most places. It can be very much taken for granted. The process of farming rice is incredibly labour intensive. It is usually done in the most poor and deprived parts of the world by people who are unwavering in their work ethic in order to feed us with this gracious grain. The rice plant seedlings are sown in paddy fields often by hand. Once the grain is ready to harvest this is again, particularly in Asia, done by hand. This is backbreaking work, often in hot climates with no shelter. The rice is laid out to dry and sometimes the outer husk needs to be removed. The rice farmer or landowner has to employ many people to oversee and produce his crop. Needless to say that the rate of pay for the worker is nowhere near the profit from the cost of the rice in the shop. This simple but intricately detailed gratitude meditation practice somehow changes absolutely everything we experience from day to day, including the act of eating rice.

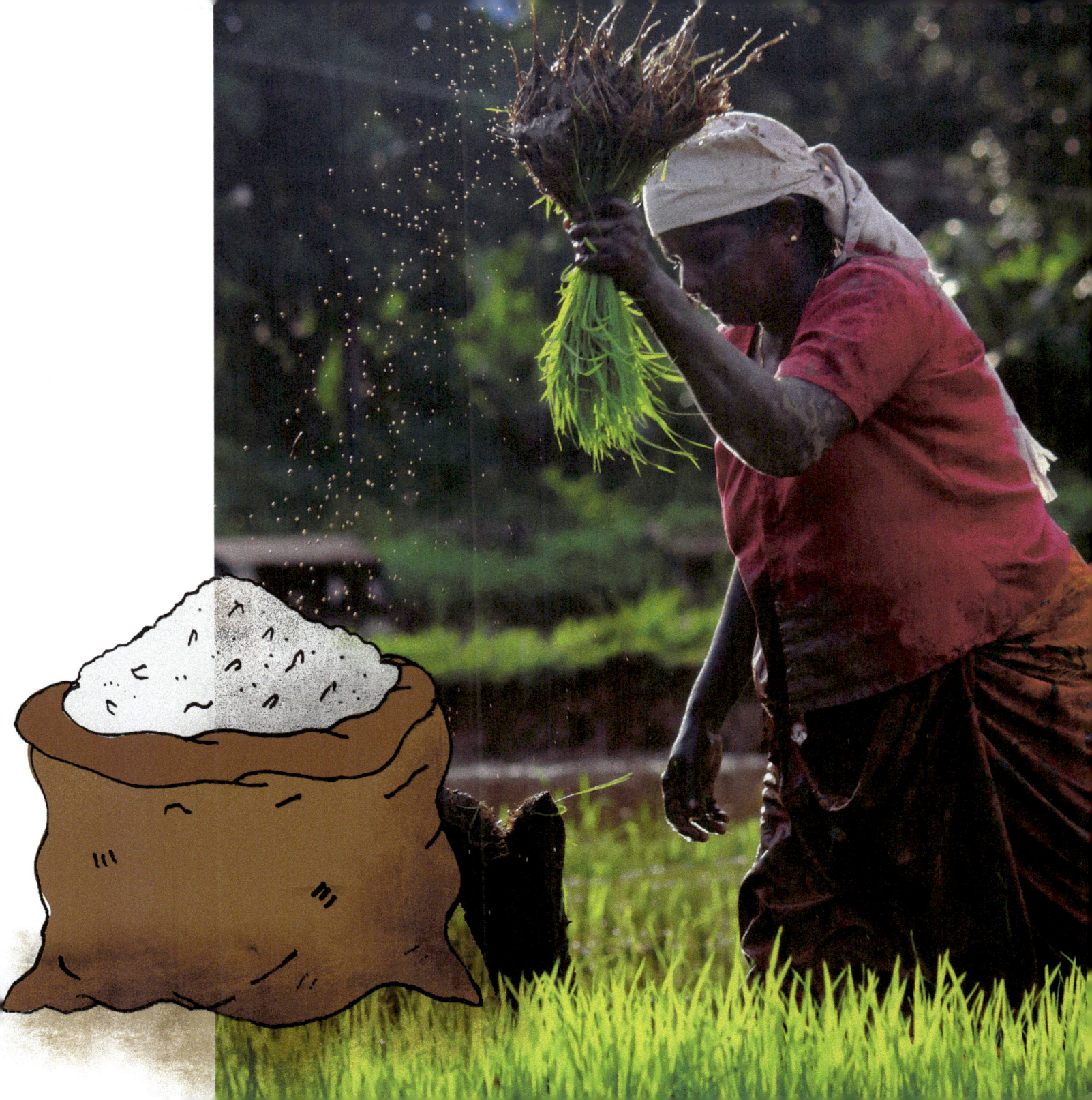

THE PRACTICE

For any seated practice make sure you are comfortable. Do not lie down as you risk falling asleep! Sit upright and be alert but relaxed. Use cushions, blankets anything you need. Have some water to hand in case you need it.

Begin by bringing to mind a bowl of freshly cooked rice - you might even want to cook some specially and have this in front of you. Notice everything about it. How many grains there must be in just this one bowl. How warm it is, the colour and how the light falls upon each and every grain. Perhaps there is steam coming from the grains. Consider how it will nourish the physical body and the effect it will have on the mind. How comforting and lovely it is to eat.

Notice how all the rice grains are the same, in shape and size, and yet each one is also subtly different somehow, unique.

Now consider where you purchased this rice. Maybe a shop or online. Consider the person who helped you to purchase this, in whatever way. They too have a home, if they're lucky they have people who love them, they eat food and navigate through life, just like you do. Send gratitude to this person. And to the people connected with them, the people who love and support them. Also to the food this person eats that sustains them so they are able to help you. You can now follow this back to the person connected to them who serves their food and so on, or continue as below.

Now consider the person who transported the rice to wherever you purchased it. Consider them in the same way as the previous person, their life, loved ones, home, food and so on. Take your time over each stage and see if you can really visualise these things and people.

Beyond this transportation we have the people who packed the rice. Who are they? Where did the rice get packaged? And what do they need to sustain and nurture them in their everyday life?

How did the rice reach the packaging people? Keep going back and back and in and in until you get all the way to the person who planted the rice seed and the people who cared for it as it grew. Consider now their life, their home, their loved ones, the food they eat, and where this comes from? How is their life? Can you send them your love and gratitude?

Sit with this for a while. Feel the enormity of it all. You may never meet these people but know that somehow you and they are linked. We are all interconnected and everything is interwoven. Just like the grains of rice. We are all the same and yet at the same time unique. Send them your deepest heartfelt gratitude and love and know that in some small way this vibration of awareness is reaching out to them. Wish all the people in your sphere of awareness well. Hold them in your awareness and in your heart for some time.

SUPPLIERS, SERVICES AND CONNECTION

The following are suppliers and teachers or services that I use and can recommend from personal experience.

Stephen Brandon ~ My primary teacher. Steve is a dedicated ayurveda and yoga practitioner who truly practices what he teaches. His depth of knowledge is second to none. If you want to get really serious, consider studying with Stephen. At the time of writing he is living in Scotland.

Devon School of Yoga ~ Duncan Hulin who founded DSY in 1989 is an inspiration. I completed all my initial teacher and yoga therapy training with him. The school offers workshops, classes, retreats and teacher trainings. If you want an authentic yoga experience do have a look. www.devonyoga.com

Tri-Dosha ~ Founded by Sunita Passi and offering ayurvedic bodywork training, beautiful ayurvedic face and body products as well as meditation and further practitioner trainings. Creative and inspiring. Sunita is also the author of the acclaimed book 'The Doctor Won't See You Now' www.tri-dosha.co.uk

Essential Ayurveda ~ An excellent small company based in the UK. Very non-commercial. High quality authentic ayurvedic products, oils, herbs and much more. www.essentialayurveda.co.uk

Wholefoods direct ~ For wholefoods online in the UK, this is an excellent supplier. www.buywholefoodsonline.co.uk

There are of course many more options. Some are listed on the 'Virginia recommends page' in the resources section of my website.

There is absolutely no substitute for supporting your local health food shop, farmers stall, market or greengrocer.

ABOUT ME

I am an ayurveda and yoga therapist, author, cyclical living advocate and eternal student of the universe.

Find me here:

Websites ~ virginiacompton.com and sattvic-soul.com

Email ~ info@virginiacompton.co.uk

Instagram and Facebook ~ virginiacomptonwellness

Chat on Telegram ~ wellness, ayurveda and yoga

SATTVIC SOUL SELF-CARE

Use this table to make notes for planning your own self-care.
It may be helpful to refer to the dosha chart on page 35 first.

My daily routine (What time do you get up, eat, sleep etc?)	**Morning:** **Afternoon:** **Evening:**
How might I begin to change my routine (if needed) so it fits more with the ayurvedic clock? (page 23)	
Foods that will nurture and balance me (page 52):	
Self-care rituals I will practice:	

Cleansing or fasting routine (one day, longer or shorter, see page 99):	
Bodymind practices (yoga, walking, breathwork, meditation):	
How can I maintain my energy and motivation?	
How will I find my people?	
Any specific health issues or things that may need addressing more. How can I begin to do this?	

BECOMING SATTVIC STARTS WITH SELF-CARE

FOR YOUR NOTES:

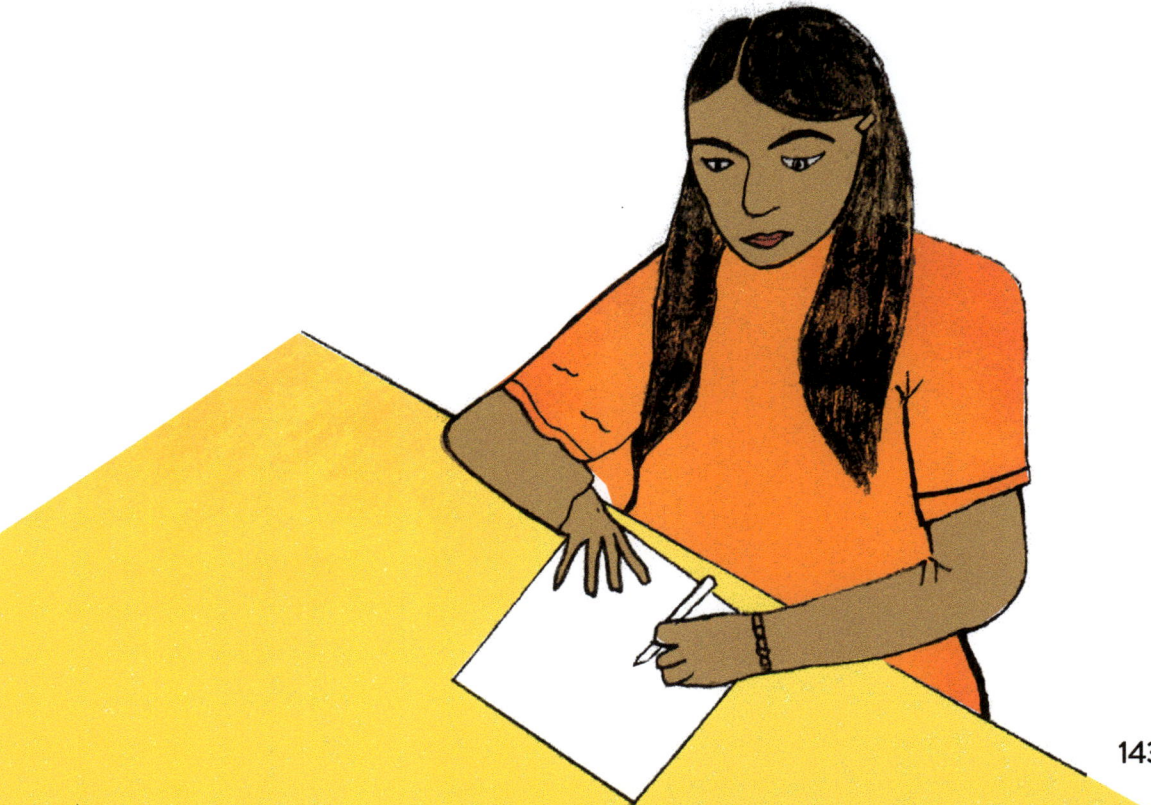

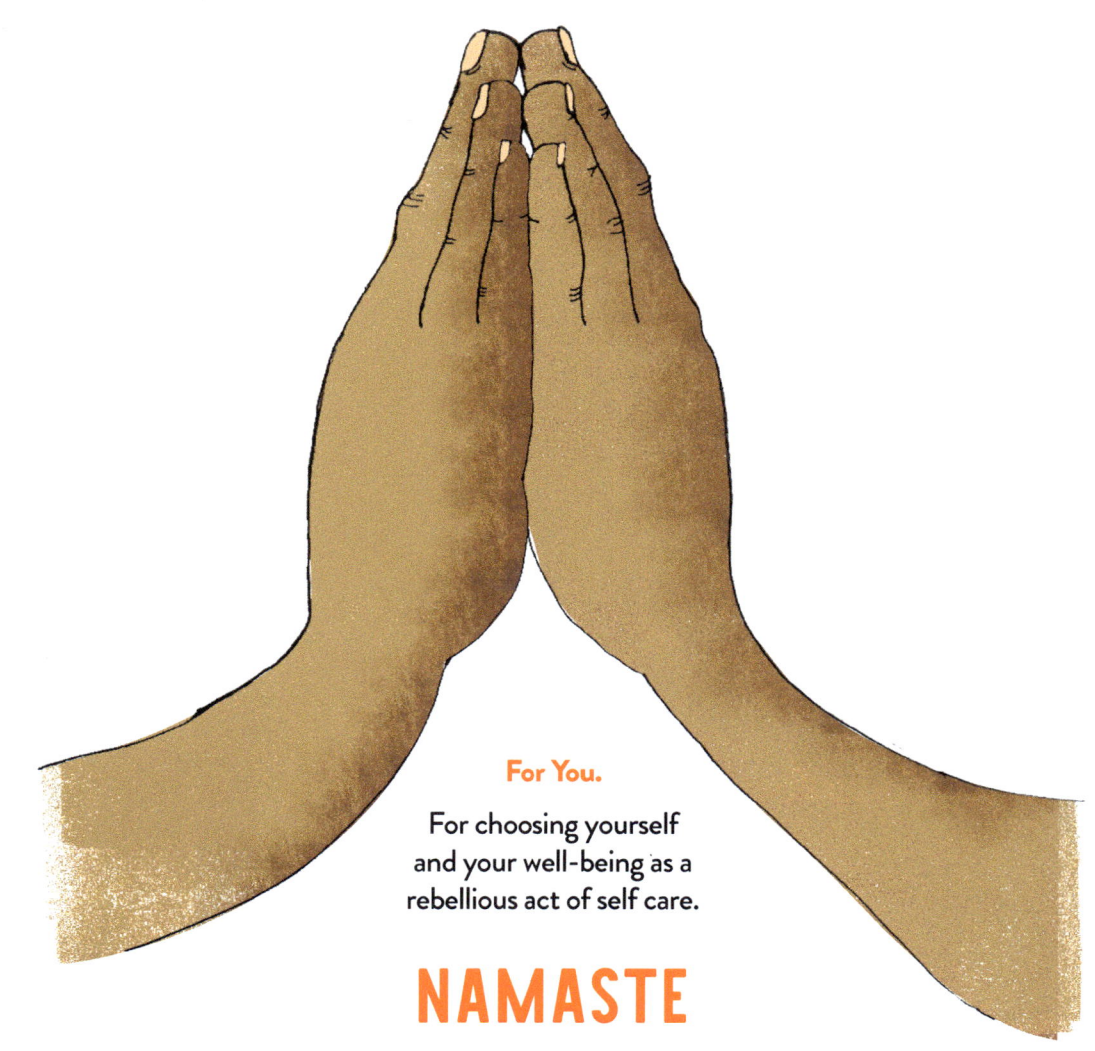

For You.

For choosing yourself
and your well-being as a
rebellious act of self care.

NAMASTE